Frozen Section Library: Lung

FROZEN SECTION LIBRARY SERIES

Philip T. Cagle, MD, Series Editor

1. Timothy Craig Allen, Philip T. Cagle: Frozen Section Library: Lung
2009   ISBN 978-0-387-09572-1

Frozen Section Library: Lung

Timothy Craig Allen, MD, JD

The University of Texas Health Science Center at Tyler, Tyler TX, USA

Philip T. Cagle, MD

Weill Cornell Medical College
The Methodist Hospital, Houston, TX, USA

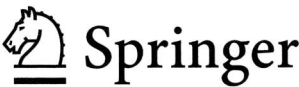

Timothy Craig Allen
Department of Pathology
The University of Texas
Health Science Center at Tyler
Tyler, TX
USA
Timothy.allen@uthct.edu

Philip T. Cagle
Department of Pathology
Weill Cornell Medical College
The Methodist Hospital
Houston, TX
USA
PCagle@tmh.tmc.edu

ISSN: xxxx
ISBN: 978-0-387-09572-1   e-ISBN: 978-0-387-09573-8
DOI: 10.1007/978-0-387-09573-8

Library of Congress Control Number: 2008928146

springer.com

To my wife, Fran, and to Caitlin and Erin
Timothy Craig Allen

To my wife, Kirsten
Philip T. Cagle

Preface

As the first volume in the Frozen Section Library Series, the Frozen Section of Lung provides a convenient, user-friendly handbook to assist in the performance of intraoperative consultations on lung specimens. This book is divided into chapters that emphasize the common questions that a pathologist must answer on frozen section examination and the pitfalls associated with those specific diagnoses. The diagnostic issues impacting immediate surgical decision-making are color-illustrated and discussed succinctly, including the well-known problems of reactive atypia versus cancer, of surgical margins, of small cell carcinoma versus non-small cell carcinoma and of primary versus metastatic cancer. The approach to benign focal lesions and wedge biopsy for diffuse lung diseases are also illustrated and discussed. We believe that this book fills a neglected niche in lung pathology and we hope that it provides useful insights for those who perform frozen sections on lung specimens.

Timothy Craig Allen, MD, JD
Philip T. Cagle, MD

Series Preface

For over 100 years, the frozen section has been utilized as a tool for the rapid diagnosis of specimens while a patient is undergoing surgery, usually under general anesthesia, as a basis for making immediate treatment decisions. Frozen section diagnosis is often a challenge for the pathologist who must render a diagnosis that has crucial import for the patient in a minimal amount of time. In addition to the need for rapid recall of differential diagnoses, there are many pitfalls and artifacts that add to the risk of frozen section diagnosis that are not present with permanent sections of fully processed tissues that can be examined in a more leisurely fashion. Despite the century-long utilization of frozen sections, most standard pathology textbooks, both general and subspecialty, largely ignore the topic of frozen sections. Few textbooks have ever focused exclusively on frozen section diagnosis and those textbooks that have done so are now out-of-date and have limited illustrations.

The Frozen Section Library series is meant to provide convenient, user-friendly handbooks for each organ system to expedite use in the rushed frozen section situation. These books are small and lightweight, copiously color-illustrated with images of actual frozen sections, highlighting pitfalls, artifacts, and differential diagnosis. The advantages of a series of organ-specific handbooks, in addition to the ease-of-use and manageable size, are that (1) a series allows more comprehensive coverage of more diagnoses, both common and rare, than a single volume that tries to highlight a limited number of diagnoses for each organ and (2) a series allows more detailed insight by permitting experienced authorities to emphasize the peculiarities of frozen section for each organ system.

As a handbook for practicing pathologists, these books will be indispensable aids to diagnosis and avoiding dangers in one of the most challenging situations that pathologists encounter. Rapid consideration of differential diagnoses and how to avoid traps caused by frozen section artifacts are emphasized in these handbooks. A series of concise, easy-to-use, well-illustrated handbooks alleviates the often frustrating and time-consuming, sometimes futile, process of searching through bulky textbooks that are unlikely to illustrate or discuss pathologic diagnoses from the perspective of frozen sections in the first place. Tables and charts will provide guidance for differential diagnosis of various histologic patterns. Touch preparations, which are used for some organs such as central nervous system or thyroid more often than others, are appropriately emphasized and illustrated according to the need for each specific organ.

This series is meant to benefit practicing surgical pathologists, both community and academic, and to pathology residents and fellows; and also to provide valuable perspectives to surgeons, surgery residents, and fellows who must rely on frozen section diagnosis by their pathologists. Most of all, we hope that this series contributes to the improved care of patients who rely on the frozen section to help guide their treatment.

Philip T. Cagle, MD
Series Editor

Contents

Chapter 1
Benign Proliferations Versus Cancer

INTRODUCTION

Frozen sections of lung cancer resection specimens (wedge resections, segmentectomies, lobectomies, and pneumonectomies) are most often performed to determine the status of surgical margins. In the majority of these specimens the diagnosis of cancer has been determined pre-operatively, but on occasion, the surgical pathologist is asked to ascertain the diagnosis of cancer at the time of frozen section, including ruling out cancer for an excised mass in the case of a localized inflammatory or other benign lesion.

While the majority of cancers and benign conditions are readily diagnosed on frozen sections of lung tissue, there are occasions when the overlap of histopathologic features, particularly when combined with frozen section artifact, make it more challenging to differentiate between benign reactive or metaplastic tissues and cancers. Since the correct diagnosis in this situation may have potential implications for immediate patient treatment, the surgical pathologist may find this diagnostic dilemma to be especially troublesome.

MEDICAL–LEGAL ISSUES WITH FROZEN SECTION

In order to render an appropriate diagnosis and therefore limit medical–legal risk, pathologists must clearly understand their role during lung frozen section, as well as the limitations of frozen section diagnosis of lung tissue. This is important to remember whether the frozen section is being performed for determination of benignity or malignancy or for any other reason, such as assessment of surgical margins. Performing a frozen section is indisputably a pressure-oriented situation. The patient remains in the operating room under anesthesia, with its inherent risks, during the entire time the pathologist is involved in rendering a frozen section diagnosis. In a timely fashion, the pathologist is generally expected to (1) orient the specimen, (2) ink margins as appropriate, (3) locate the lesion or

T.C. Allen, P.T. Cagle, *Frozen Section Library: Lung*,
Frozen Section Library 1, DOI 10.1007/978-0-387-09573-8_1,
© Springer Science+Business Media, LLC 2009

lesions present, (4) decide what tissue to sample, (5) sometimes cut and stain the section and prepare the slide, (6) examine the slide in a less reliable and less thorough manner than is possible with permanent section, (7) render a diagnosis, and (8) communicate that diagnosis to the surgeon who will then determine the appropriate action to be taken based, in large part if not almost entirely, on the pathologist's diagnosis.

In performing the frozen section, a pathologist has a legal duty to provide care conforming to the standard of care. The pathologist must possess and apply the knowledge and use the amount of care that a reasonably well-qualified pathologist would use under similar circumstances. In the event of a lawsuit based on a frozen section diagnosis, whether the pathologist acted with reasonable care and diligence under the specific circumstances of that frozen section is determined, generally by a jury, based on testimony from expert witnesses who present to the court evidence of the applicable standard of care and opinions as to whether that standard was breached under the circumstances. Given the frequently extreme differences in treatment choices from which the surgeon chooses based on the frozen section diagnosis, it is imperative that the diagnosis of malignancy be made only when the criteria for that diagnosis are clearly present at frozen section. As a general rule, the pathologist at frozen section should err on the side of caution, and if doubt exists, await complete and thorough examination of the specimen by permanent sections before making a diagnosis.

PROCESSES WITH REACTIVE ATYPIA

Reactive epithelial atypia, metaplastic epithelium, reactive fibroblasts, and reactive endothelial cells may mimic neoplastic cells, particularly when their apparent size and shape are distorted by frozen section artifact. Reactive atypia may result in increased cellularity, enlarged nuclei, hyperchromatic nuclei, and mitoses that in some cases resemble features of malignant cells. Metaplasia results in the presence of proliferating cells that are not normally seen in the specific location (lining airways, alveoli or residual cystic spaces in honey-comb lung) so that they may suggest a neoplastic proliferation. Specific cell types that may display reactive or metaplastic changes that sometimes mimic neoplastic cells are listed in Table 1.1.

Processes that may produce reactive or metaplastic cells are listed in Table 1.2 along with their associated histopathologic features. These associated histopathologic features may provide clues to the reactive or metaplastic nature of the cells in frozen sections, but many

TABLE 1.1. Specific pulmonary cell types potentially displaying reactive atypia and/or metaplasia

Endothelial cells: Reactive atypia (Figs. 1.1 and 1.2)

Fibroblasts: Reactive atypia (Figs. 1.3 and 1.4)

Bronchial epithelium: Reactive atypia; squamous metaplasia; goblet cell (mucinous) metaplasia (Fig. 1.5)

Bronchiolar epithelium: Reactive atypia; goblet cell (mucinous) metaplasia; squamous metaplasia (Fig. 1.6)

Alveolar epithelium: Hyperplasia with or without reactive atypia including intranuclear inclusions; cuboidal metaplasia; bronchiolar metaplasia; goblet cell (mucinous) metaplasia; squamous metaplasia (Figs. 1.7, 1.8, 1.9, 1.10)

TABLE 1.2. Conditions Associated with Reactive and Metaplastic Alveolar Epithelium

Condition	Other prominent features
Diffuse alveolar damage	Hyaline membranes lining alveoli; interstitial granulation tissue; may include intra-alveolar edema or hemorrhage; may include viral inclusions or other findings correlating with specific etiologies
Acute fibrinous and organizing pneumonia	Intra-alveolar fibrinous exudates; intra-alveolar granulation tissue; may include viral inclusions or other findings correlating with specific etiologies
Organizing pneumonia	Intra-alveolar granulation tissue; granulation tissue may extend into bronchioles; may include viral inclusions, aspirated material, granulomas or other findings correlating with specific etiologies
Interstitial pneumonia	Interstitial cellular infiltrates (lymphocytes, plasma cells, etc.); may also include interstitial fibrosis (collagen, granulation tissue); may include viral inclusions, granulomas, etc., correlating with specific etiologies
Interstitial fibrosis/Honey-comb lung	Interstitial collagen; obliteration of architecture by collagen with residual cystic spaces; may include lymphoid aggregates; may include granulomas, asbestos bodies, etc., correlating with specific etiologies

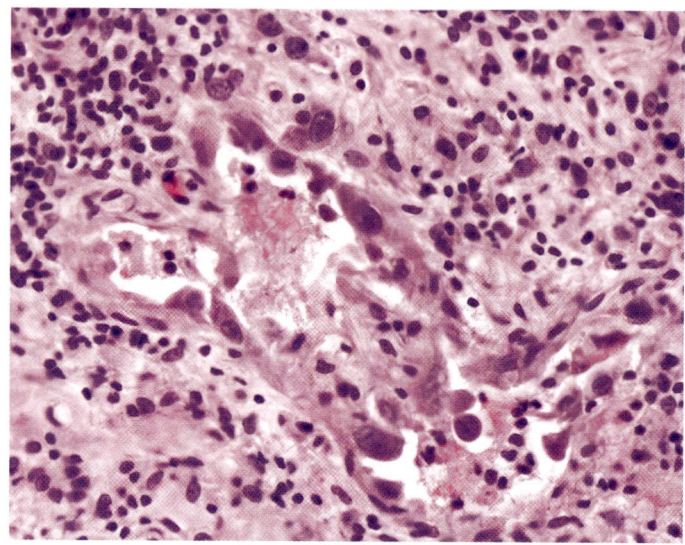

FIGURE 1.1. Reactive endothelial cells (enlarged cuboidal-to-polygonal cells with enlarged nuclei and prominent nucleoli) line a vascular space in a frozen section of a wedge biopsy of organizing pneumonia. Additional apparent enlargement and distortion of the reactive endothelial cells and their nuclei is the result of frozen section artifact. Focally, there are red blood cells and fibrin within the lumen which identifies this structure as a blood vessel.

of these features can also be seen in frozen sections containing cancers. For example, organizing pneumonia and interstitial lymphocytic infiltrates may be seen as a peri-tumoral response or post-obstructive change associated with cancers. Therefore, associated histopathologic features must be interpreted within the overall context.

HISTOLOGIC FEATURES THAT OVERLAP BETWEEN BENIGN REACTIVE PROLIFERATIONS AND CANCER

Histopathologic features of benign reactive proliferations that may mimic the histopathologic features associated with cancers are listed in Table 1.3. These overlapping features are well-recognized as potential causes of diagnostic difficulty in permanent histologic sections. However, they may be even more indistinguishable in frozen sections where cells may appear enlarged and distorted by artifact, compounding the difficulty in interpretation.

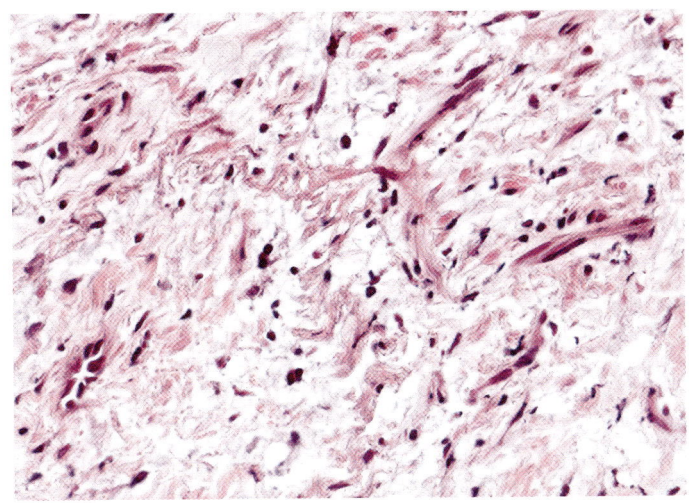

FIGURE 1.2. The reactive endothelial cells lining capillaries appear as cuboidal-to-elongate cells with dark-staining enlarged nuclei within a fibroblastic stroma in this frozen section of a fibrotic pulmonary process. Frozen section artifact distorts the capillary lumens and further obscures the details of the endothelial cells, enhancing their resemblance to atypical epithelial cells. These features may sometimes be suggestive of invasive glands and cords of cells of a carcinoma.

DIFFERENTIATION OF BENIGN REACTIVE PROLIFERATIONS FROM MALIGNANCY ON FROZEN SECTION

Histopathologic findings that may help differentiate between reactive proliferations and cancers are provided in Table 1.4. To avoid potential pitfalls, the pathologist should first be cognizant that reactive atypia or metaplasia may occasionally resemble malignancy in some lung specimens and that the similarity can be exacerbated by the added artifacts of frozen section. Examination of the gross specimen is often helpful: recognition that the disease is grossly a diffuse inflammatory process or otherwise lacks gross features of a neoplasm puts the microscopic observations in a different context. However, many cancers will be grossly surrounded by peri-tumoral or post-obstructive inflammation or pneumonia and, while most of these will be recognizable grossly as neoplasms, gross observations may occasionally be equivocal. Bronchioloalveolar carcinomas may rarely present as a "pneumonic" process or may be grossly difficult to identify because the parenchymal architecture is preserved.

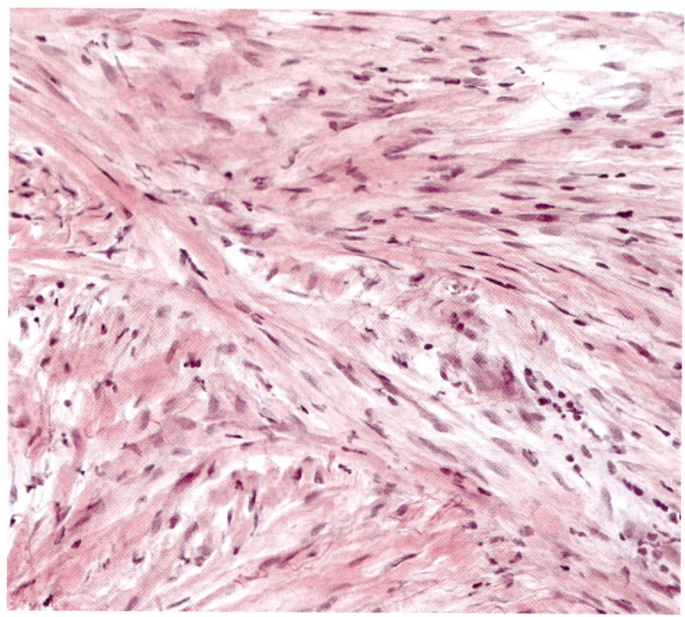

FIGURE 1.3. Low-power view of frozen section of an active pulmonary fibrotic process shows increased cellularity due to proliferating fibroblasts. In addition to the increased cellularity, some fibroblasts show enlarged elongate nuclei with further distortion of nuclear features by frozen section artifact. These features may sometimes be worrisome for a spindle cell malignancy.

Clinical information and observations of the surgeon also help to put a specimen into proper context. As noted above, since most lung cancers are diagnosed prior to surgery, if a frozen section is being carried out to confirm malignancy, there is obviously a clinical/surgical question about the diagnosis. However, it is helpful to know what clinical diagnosis is favored and to confirm that one is dealing with a mass and not a diffuse process. Information on requisition slips may not always be complete, so direct verbal communication with the surgeon is important. Orienting the specimen and directing the pathologist to the area of most concern by placing a marking suture are two ways the surgeon can facilitate an accurate diagnosis.

Assessment of the histologic context in which cytologically atypical cells are present is very helpful in determining if a process is benign reactive proliferation or carcinoma. A reactive process is favored when the volume of organizing or mature fibrosis and

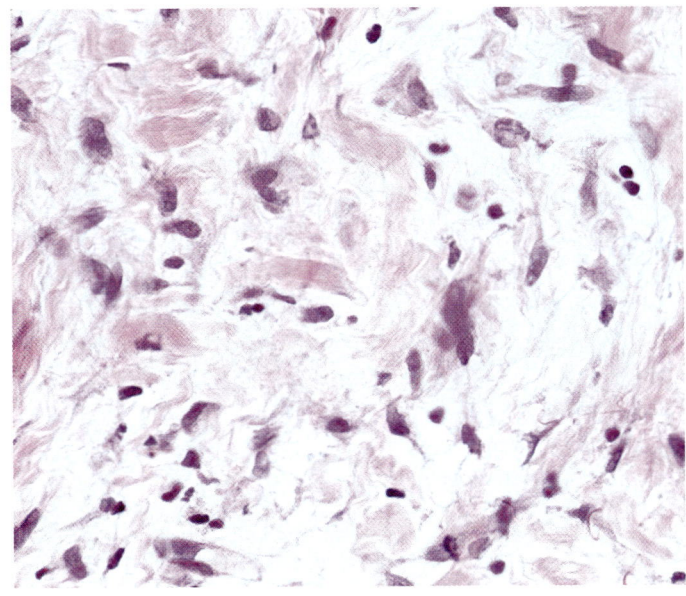

FIGURE 1.4. Higher-power view shows enlarged, variably irregular nuclei of reactive fibroblasts in a frozen section of pulmonary granulation tissue. Some fibroblasts have nucleoli.

inflammation are disproportionate to the volume of atypical cells and extend substantially beyond the atypical cells into surrounding tissues. Uniform cytologic atypia, as opposed to variable cytologic atypia mixed with less atypical or normal cells, favors malignancy. However, none of these observations is foolproof since, for example, only a few malignant cells may be present in a biopsy that otherwise shows inflammation or fibrosis. None of these features should be judged outside of its overall context. If, after applying these criteria, the histologic features remain equivocal, it is best to err on the side of caution and defer the diagnosis for permanent sections.

DIFFERENTIATION OF TYPE II PNEUMOCYTE HYPERPLASIA FROM BRONCHIOLOALVEOLAR PATTERN OF ADENOCARCINOMA

Distinguishing reactive type II pneumocyte hyperplasia from bronchioloalveolar pattern of carcinoma can be difficult on frozen section. Several features that may be helpful in distinguishing

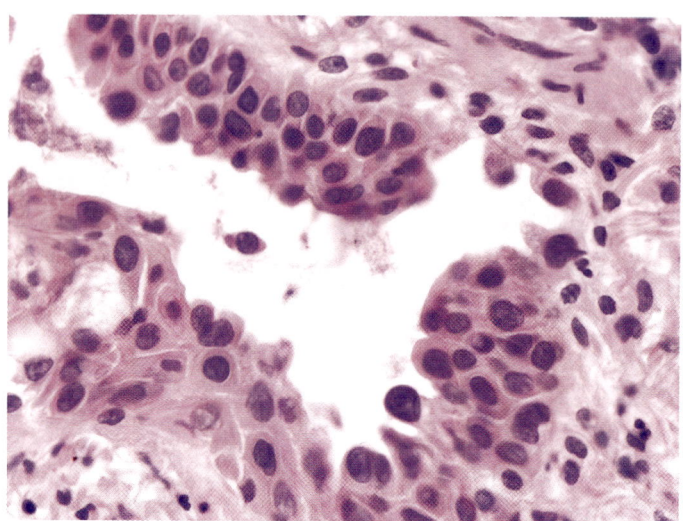

FIGURE 1.5. Frozen section of squamous metaplasia of bronchial epithelium in an inflammatory process. In addition to having squamous features, the epithelial cells show reactive atypia including enlarged, hyperchromatic nuclei with mild variation in size and shape which is further magnified by frozen section artifact.

reactive atypia from bronchioloalveolar pattern of carcinoma on frozen section are summarized in Table 1.5. Once again, these features should not be interpreted individually outside of the overall context and if the histologic features remain ambiguous, it is best to defer to permanent sections.

MEGAKARYOCYTES

Megakaryocytes (Fig. 1.29) within pulmonary alveolar capillaries are frequently seen in lung tissue and are found in increased numbers in various conditions such as disseminated intravascular coagulation, metastatic pulmonary malignancies, burn injury, and

→

FIGURE 1.7 High-power view of frozen section showing focus of reactive hyperplastic type II pneumocytes in organizing acute lung injury. Enlarged alveolar epithelial cells display enlarged nuclei with moderate variability in size and shape and occasional nucleoli.

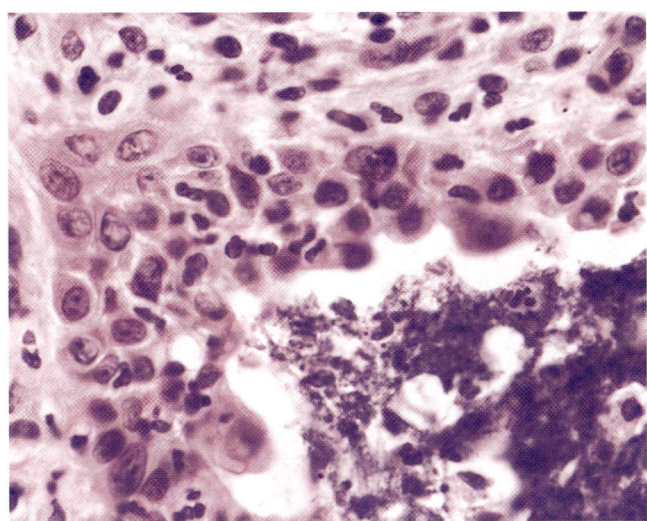

FIGURE 1.6. Squamous metaplasia with reactive changes of bronchiolar epithelium in a frozen section of organizing acute lung injury. The metaplastic epithelium displays enlarged nuclei that vary from dark to vesicular with nucleoli, features that may be potentially worrisome for carcinoma. The bronchiolar lumen contains necroinflammatory debris.

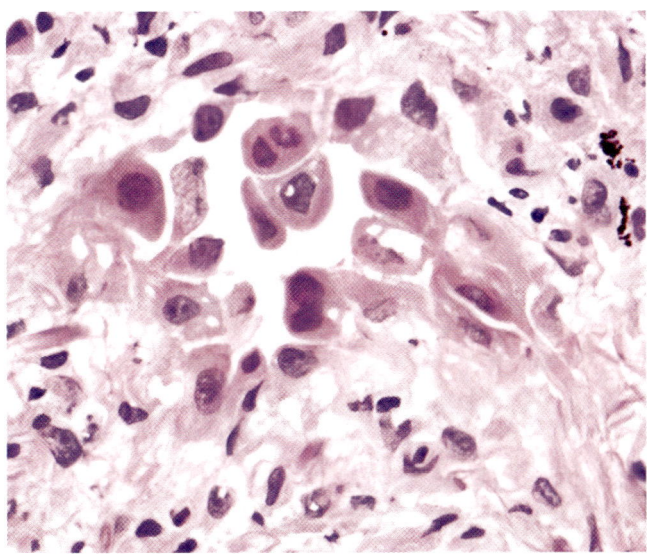

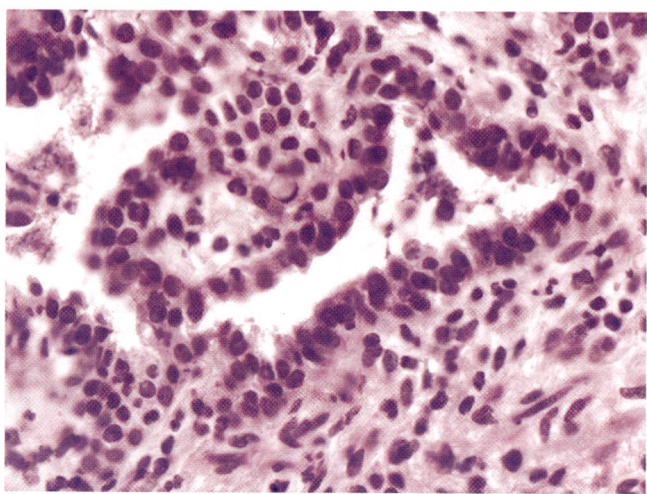

FIGURE 1.8. High-power view of reactive type II pneumocyte hyperplasia in a frozen section of an inflammatory fibrotic pulmonary lesion. The nuclei are mildly enlarged and dark with occasional small intranuclear inclusions. These features may potentially suggest an adenocarcinoma or bronchioloalveolar carcinoma.

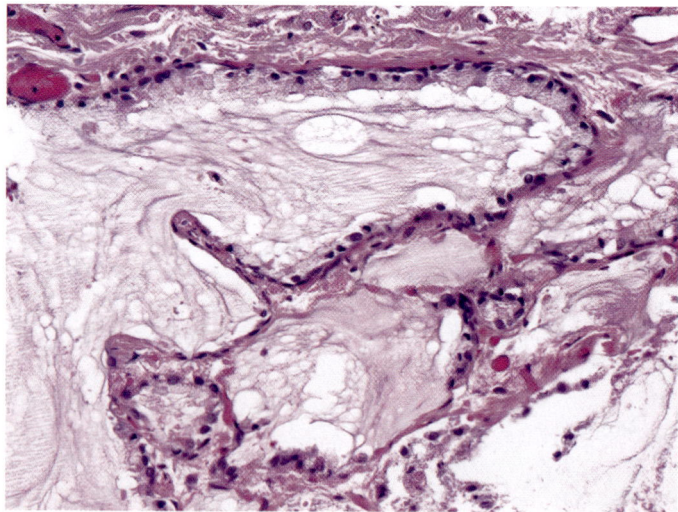

FIGURE 1.9. Low-power view shows area of metaplastic mucin-producing goblet cells lining residual airspaces in organizing diffuse alveolar damage.

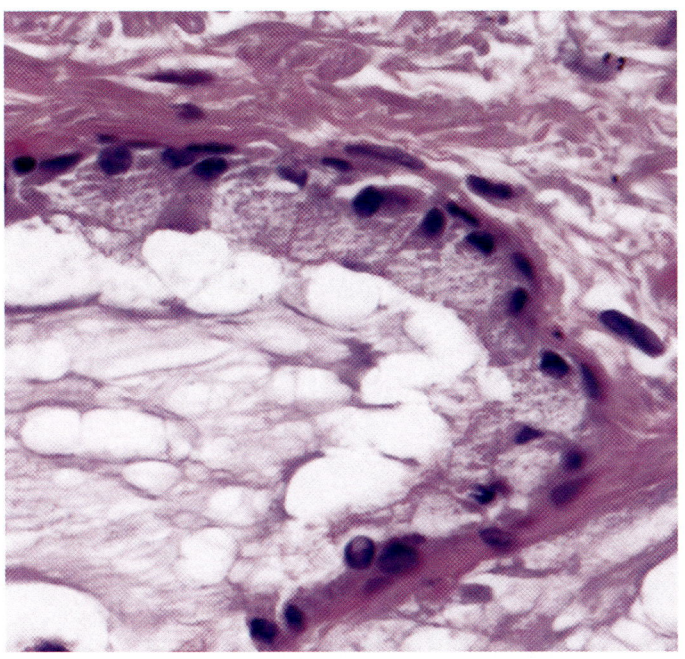

FIGURE 1.10. High-power view shows that the metaplastic goblet cells have bland, basal nuclei but lack the cytologic atypia of mucinous adenocarcinoma on the one hand and the monotonous uniformity of cells of bronchioloalveolar carcinoma on the other.

acute respiratory distress syndrome. Pulmonary megakaryocytes may occasionally be found on frozen section and care must be taken not to over-diagnose them. The large, dark, multilobated nucleus of a pulmonary megakaryocyte may mimic a neoplastic cell or a cell with a viral inclusion. Their location within septal capillaries and their distribution as scattered single cells help identify them as megakaryocytes.

◄────────────────────────────────────

FIGURE 1.9 *Continued* These metaplastic cells lining airspaces with walls thickened by fibrosis may resemble mucinous adenocarcinoma or mucinous bronchioloalveolar carcinoma.

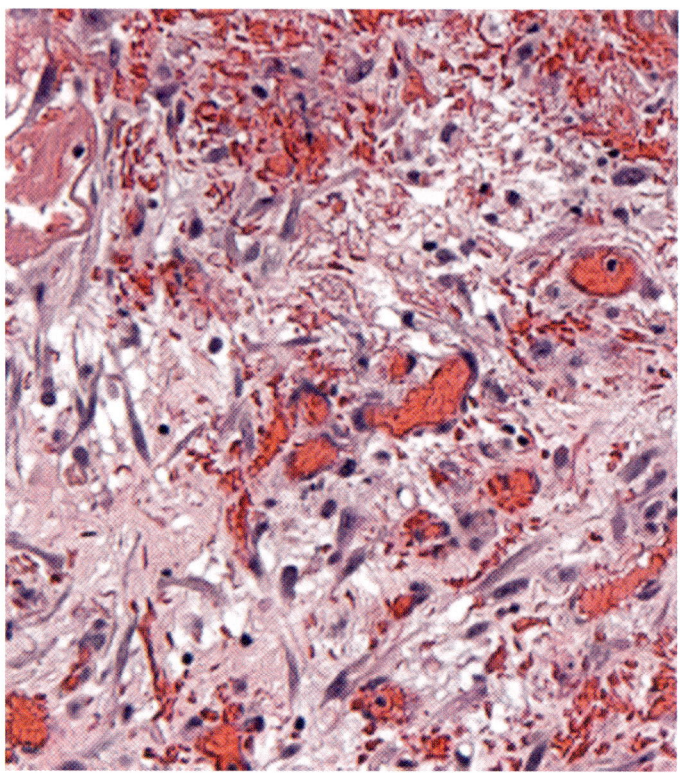

FIGURE 1.11. Medium-power view of reactive fibroblasts in organizing pneumonia shows increased cellularity. Frozen artifact obscures cytologic details making interpretation of the reactive cells more difficult.

TABLE 1.3. Histopatholgic features of benign reactive proliferations that may mimic histopathologic features of cancers

Increased cellularity (increased numbers of cells; crowding of cells) (Fig. 1.11)
Altered tissue architecture (Fig. 1.12):
   Features adjacent to the proliferating cells such as fibrosis;
   Apparent stratification or piling up of proliferating cells;
   Groups, nests or lining of reactive or metaplastic cells that are not normally
   observed in the specific location usually lining airways, alveoli or residual
   cysts of honey-comb lung
Enlarged overall cell size
Enlarged nuclear size

TABLE 1.3. *Continued*

Hyperchromatic nuclei
Prominent nucleoli (Fig. 1.13)
Mitoses (Fig. 1.14)
Intra-nuclear inclusions (Fig. 1.15)
Necrosis (Fig. 1.16)
Reactive cells within granulation tissue, organizing pneumonia, etc., may mimic invasive malignant cells with desmoplastic reaction (Fig. 1.17)

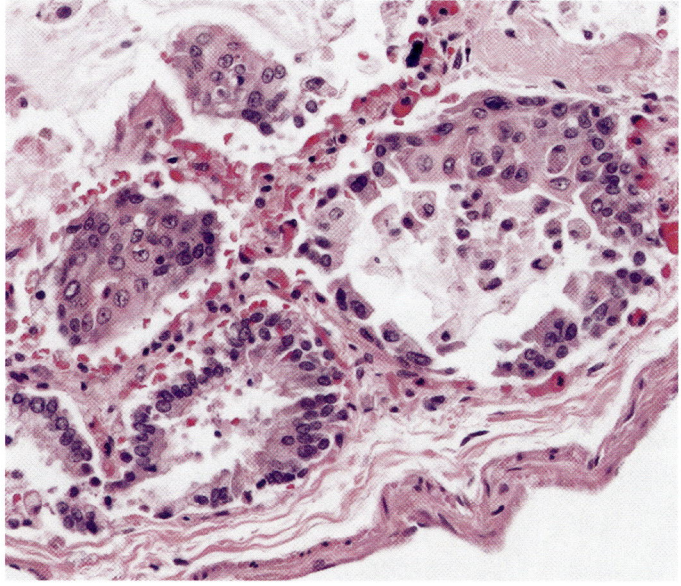

FIGURE 1.12. Medium-power view of organizing acute lung injury shows nests of metaplastic squamous cells and stratified metaplastic cells lining residual airspaces.

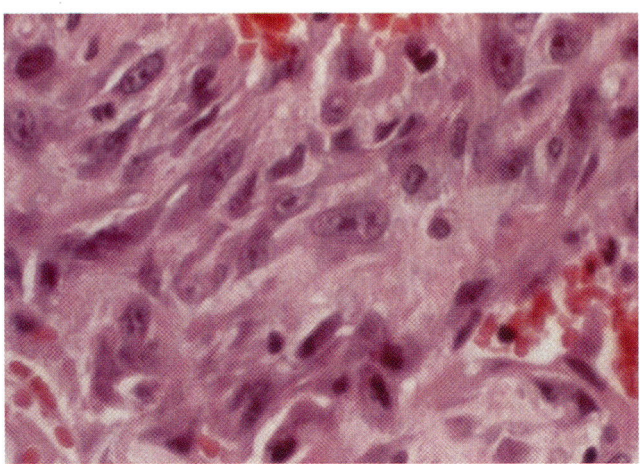

FIGURE 1.13. High-power view shows reactive fibroblasts in organizing acute lung injury with enlarged vesicular nuclei and prominent nucleoli.

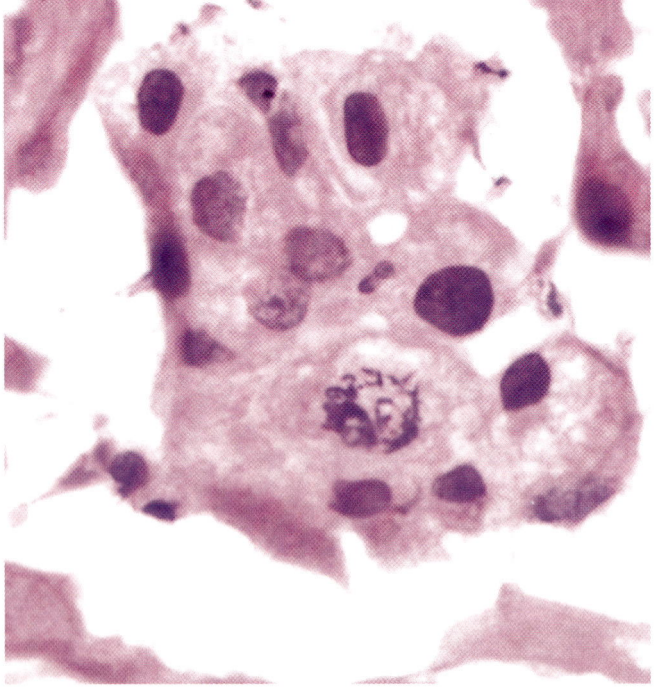

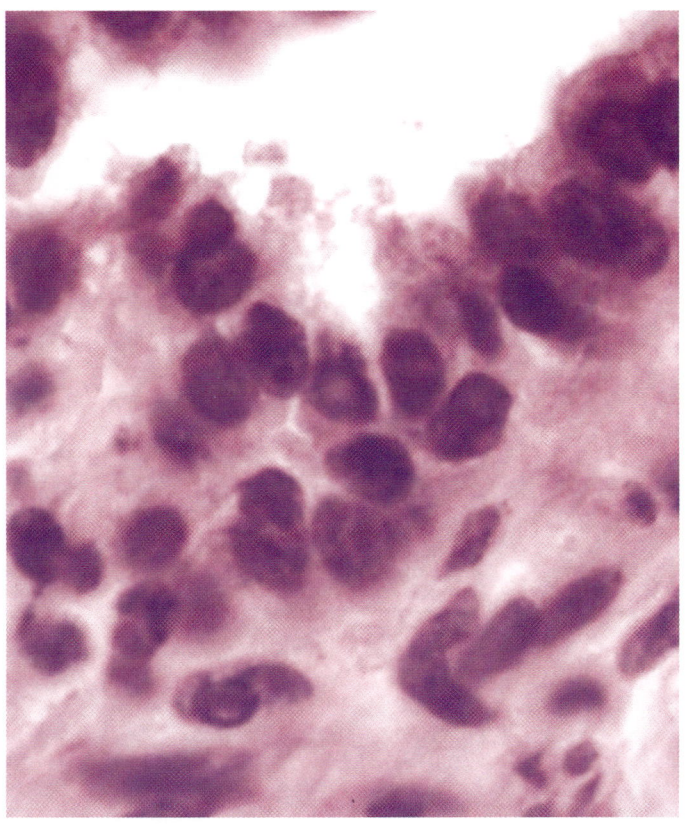

FIGURE 1.15. High-power view shows a reactive type II pneumocyte with a small intranuclear inclusion.

◄—————————————————————————————————

FIGURE 1.14. High-power view shows a cluster of reactive cells in organizing pneumonia, including a mitotic figure.

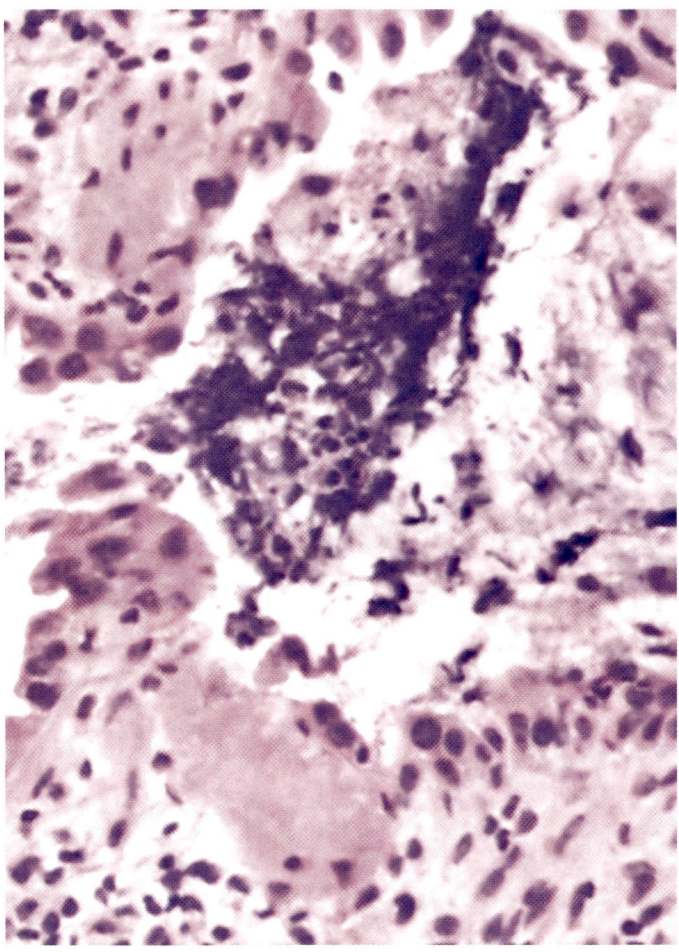

FIGURE 1.16. Medium-power view of an organizing acute lung injury with necrosis in an airspace lined by reactive epithelial cells.

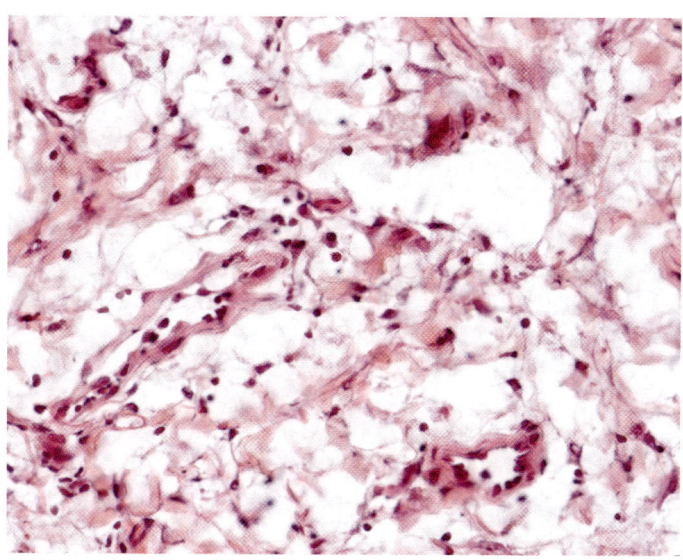

FIGURE 1.17. Small vessels lined by reactive endothelial cells and further distorted by frozen section artifact are present within loose granulation tissue of organizing acute lung injury and may resemble small glands infiltrating a desmoplastic stroma.

TABLE 1.4. Histologic features that favor reactive proliferations or cancers (Figures 1-18 through 1-25)

Favors benign reactive proliferation	Favors cancer
Atypia relatively mild and proportionate to surrounding inflammatory or fibrotic process; enlarged nuclei maintain normal contours; smooth nuclear borders	Severe cytologic atypia that in absence of or disproportionate to surrounding inflammatory or fibrotic process; enlarged nuclei with irregular nuclear contours; sharp angulated nuclear borders
Cytoplasm is proportionately increased in relation to enlarged nucleus or cell	High nucleus–cytoplasm ratio
Spectrum of cytologic atypia is present with atypical cells blending with less atypical cells and normal cells	All cells in the population show significant cytologic pleomorphism
Normal mitoses	Abnormal mitoses

TABLE 1.4. *Continued*

Favors benign reactive proliferation	Favors cancer
Intra-nuclear inclusions absent or few	Intra-nuclear inclusions prominent and multiple
Reactive cells line preserved architecture or simple cystic spaces	Malignant cells line complex architecture: variably sized glands; cribriform pattern; papillary structures with cores
Well-demarcated margins of groups of reactive cells	Irregular borders with infiltrative groups of malignant cells or individual malignant cells
Inflammation, fibrosis, and/or parenchymal damage extends beyond cells with reactive atypia	Inflammation and fibrosis limited to area in and immediately adjacent to malignant cells

TABLE 1.5. Reactive Atypia of type II Pneumocytes Versus Bronchioloalveolar Carcinoma

Reactive atypia	Bronchioloalveolar carcinoma
Associated with parenchymal damage or fibrosis larger than area of epithelial atypia	Desmoplasia limited to septa lined by neoplastic cells
Mixed cell types	Uniformity of cell type
Mixed degrees of cytologic atypia	Uniformity of cytologic atypia
Rare, small intranuclear inclusions	Frequent, large intranuclear inclusions
Cilia may be present	Cilia not present
Blends into adjacent epithelium	Abrupt demarcation from adjacent epithelium
Attached to septa in single row	Projecting tufts or buds; aerogenous spread

⟶

FIGURE 1.19. At low power, the volume of fibrosis and inflammation is disproportionately greater than the number of atypical reactive cells. While not definitive for a benign process, this increased ratio of fibrosis and inflammation to reactive epithelial cells is typical of a non-neoplastic process.

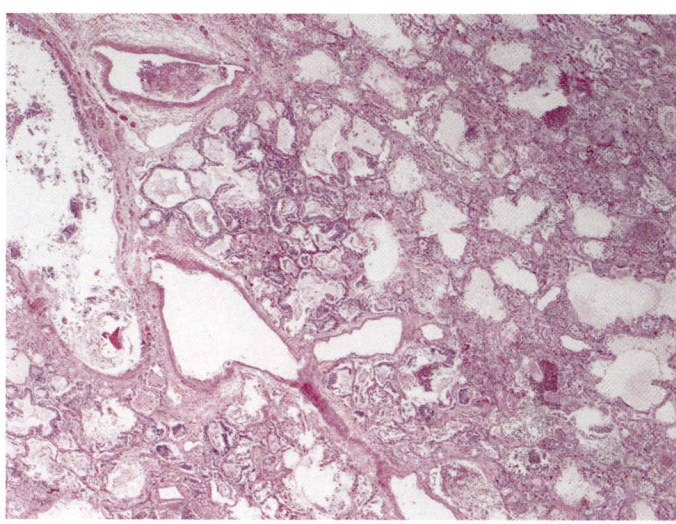

FIGURE 1.18. At low power, the area of alveolar spaces lined by metaplastic epithelium is surrounded by much more extensive acute lung injury, with hyaline membranes, fibrinous exudates, and early organization. Observation power permits interpretation of the metaplastic epithelium within the context of the background of acute lung injury.

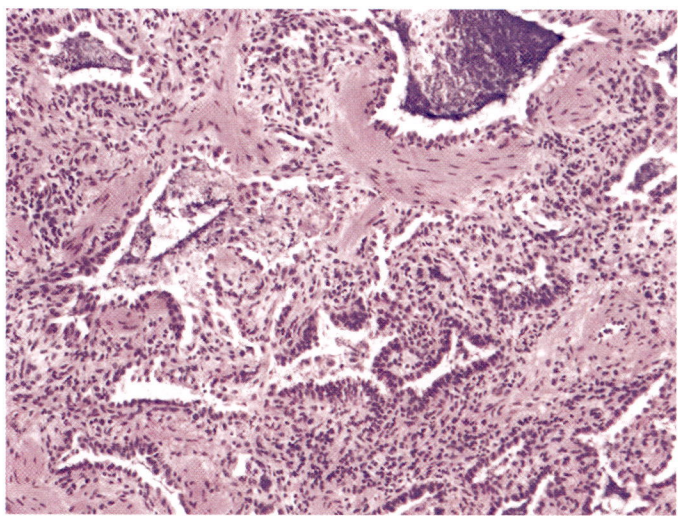

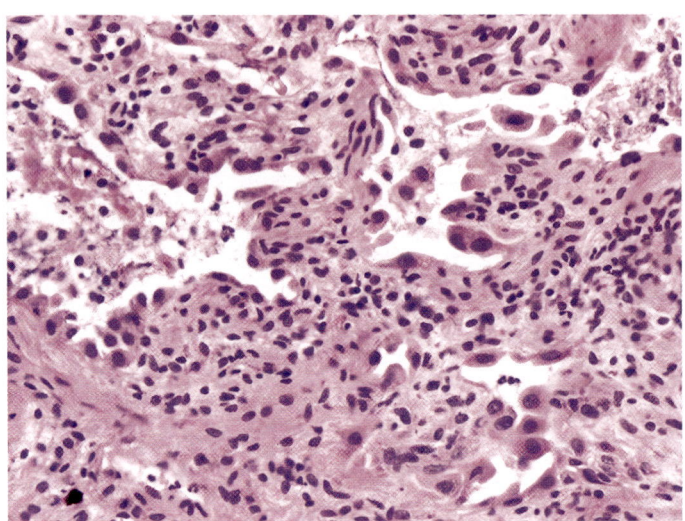

FIGURE 1.20. At medium power, epithelial cells of varying size and varying shape (flat-to-cuboidal-to-low columnar) intermingle along alveolar septa that are thickened with edema, inflammatory cells, and fibrosis. Enlarged nuclei are relatively proportionate to enlarged cells with increased cytoplasm. This variation in degree of cytologic atypia is typical of a reactive process.

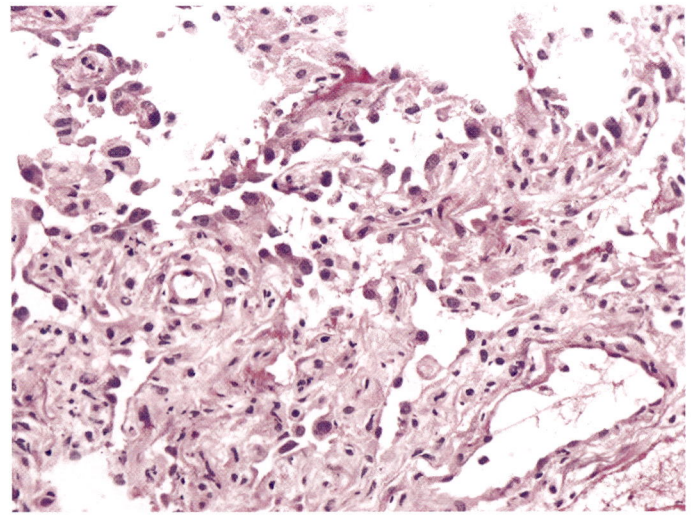

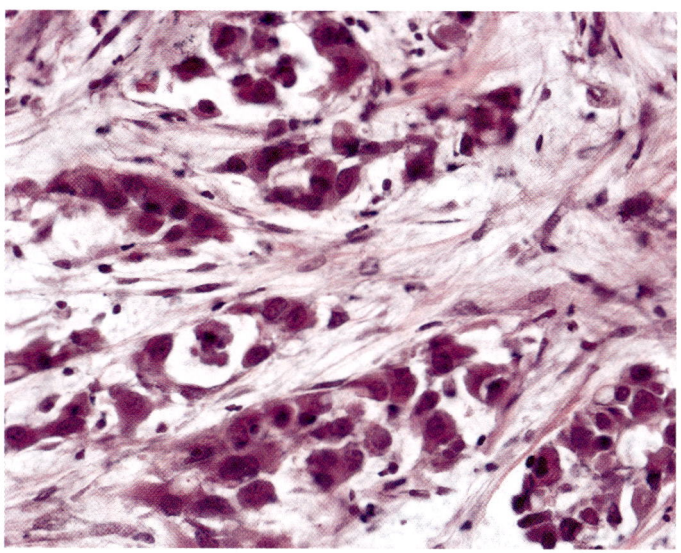

FIGURE 1.22. All of the epithelial cells in this adenocarcinoma uniformly show significant cytologic atypia and high nuclear–cytoplasmic ratios. This is in contrast to the wide range of normal or near-normal cells mixed with cells with differing degrees of cytologic atypia characteristic of a reactive process.

FIGURE 1.21. Although some atypical cells stand out, nearly normal epithelial cells blend with cuboidal/low columnar cells with enlarged nuclei and prominent nucleoli in this case of organizing pneumonia.

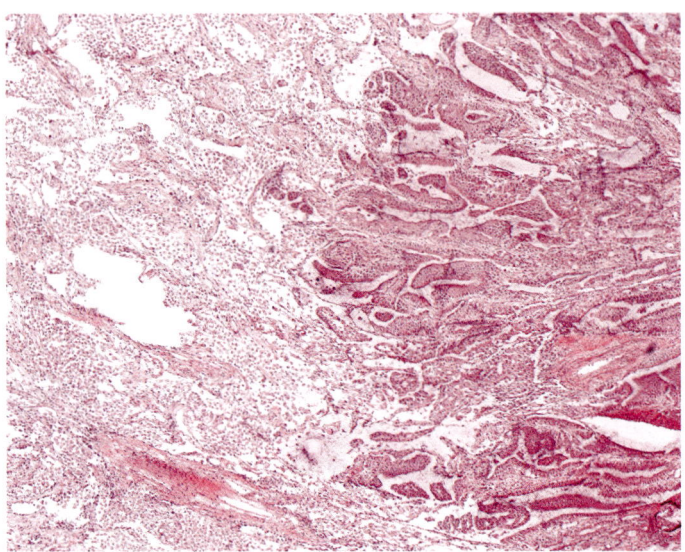

FIGURE 1.23. Low-power view shows edge of adenocarcinoma without extension of fibrosis or significant inflammation into adjacent lung parenchyma. The atypical epithelial proliferation of the cancer is disproportionate to the amount of surrounding fibrosis and inflammation. There are abundant macrophages within the adjacent alveolar spaces uninvolved by the cancer.

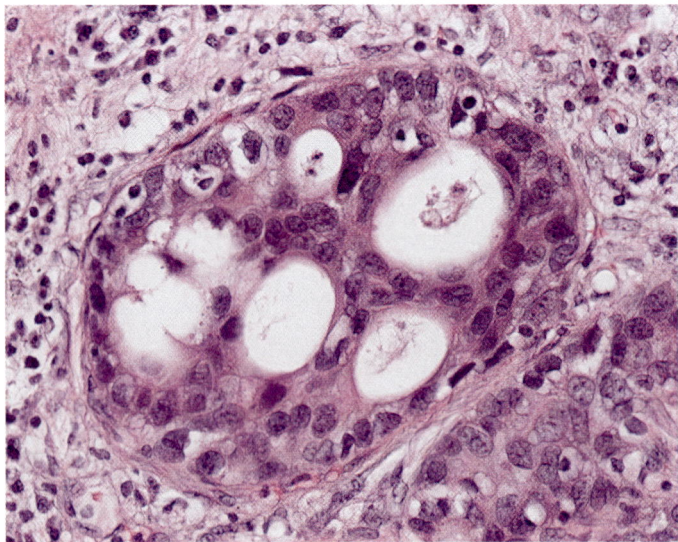

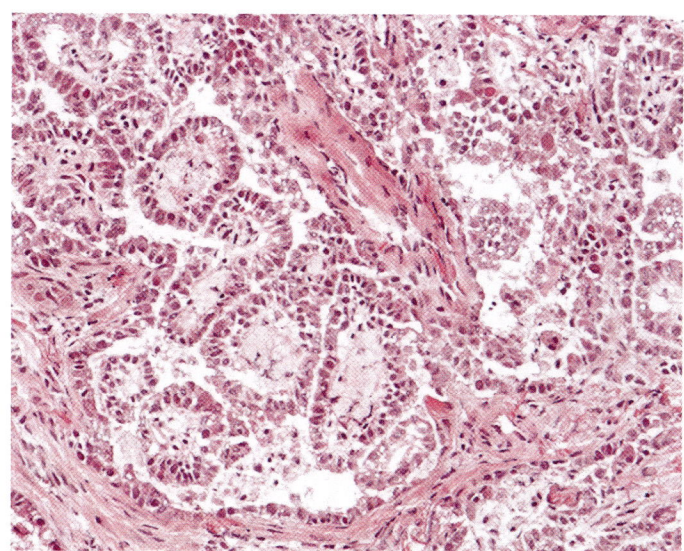

FIGURE 1.25. Papillary structures with fibrovascular cores lined by epithelial cells that uniformly exhibit cytologic pleomorphism and high nucleus–cytoplasm ratio obviously represent a papillary adenocarcinoma of the lung.

◄──

FIGURE 1.24. Cribriform architecture composed of epithelial cells, all of which uniformly show cytologic pleomorphism and high nucleus–cytoplasm ratio, is obviously malignant.

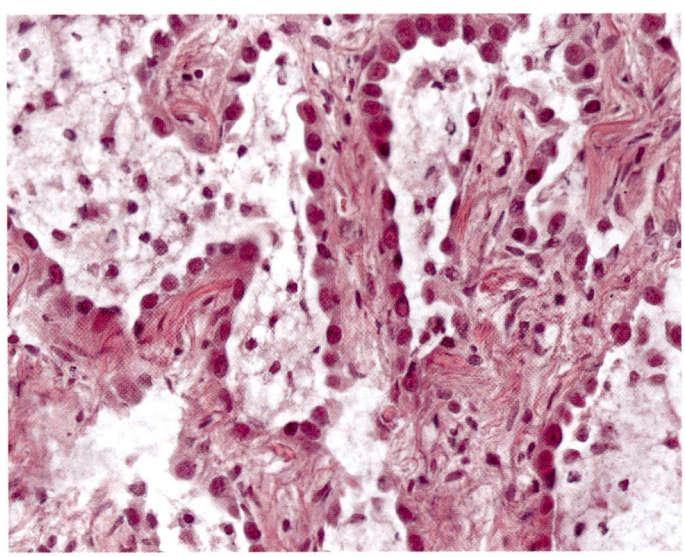

FIGURE 1.26. The epithelial cells lining these thickened alveolar septa uniformly display approximately the same amount of cytologic pleomorphism. This is bronchioloalveolar carcinoma.

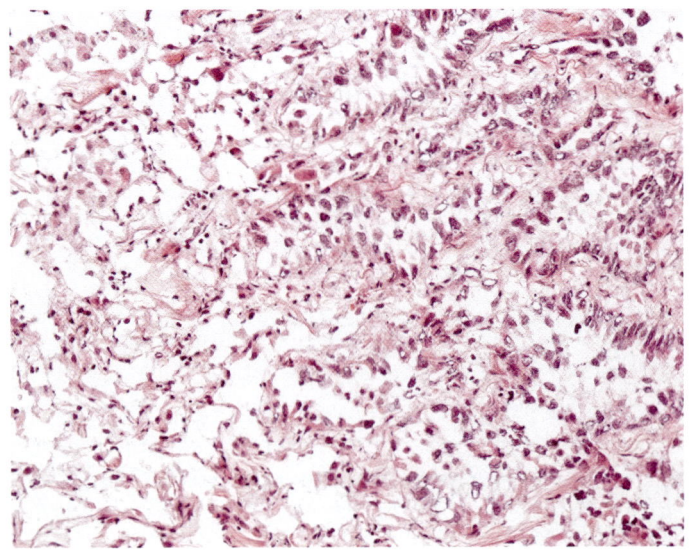

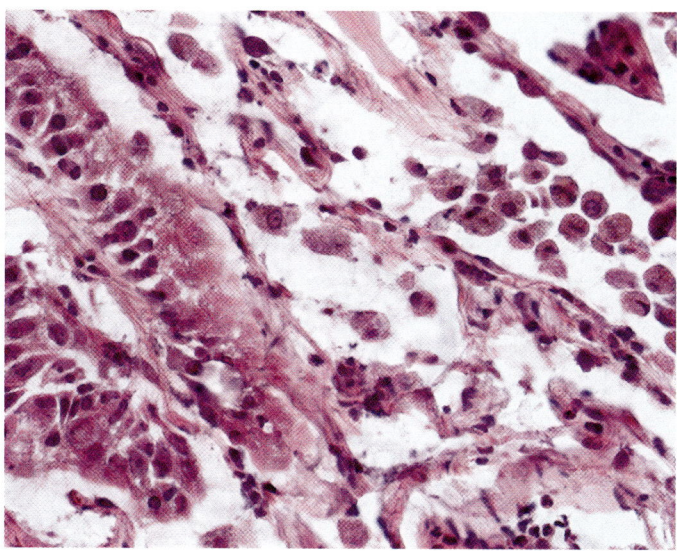

FIGURE 1.28. High-power view shows the same features as shown in Fig. 1.27 at closer view. The malignant cells are comparatively homogeneous: they are all columnar with cytologic pleomorphism and high nucleus–cytoplasm ratio consistently present in all of the malignant cells. There is an abrupt boundary between the malignant cells growing along the alveolar septa and the adjacent septa lined by an uneven mixture of normal-to-reactive epithelial cells.

FIGURE 1.27. Medium-power view shows sharp demarcation between the malignant cells lining fibrotic alveolar septa and thin alveolar septa lined by an admixture of normal-to-reactive epithelial cells.

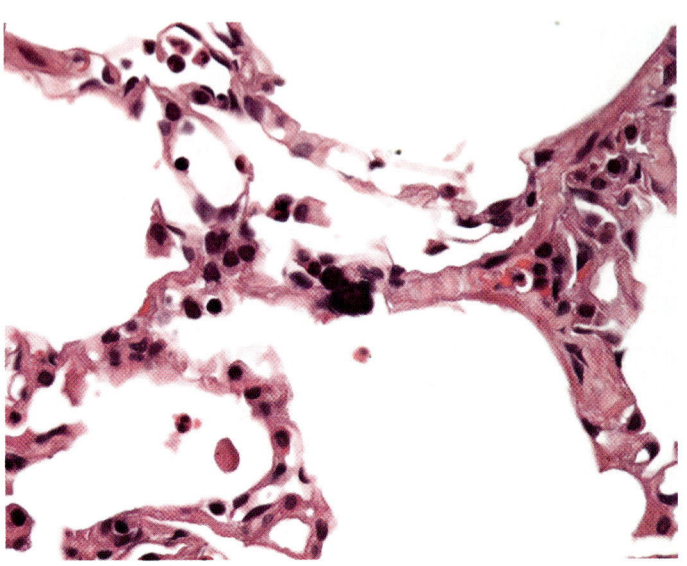

FIGURE 1.29. A megakaryocyte within an alveolar capillary appears as a large, irregularly shaped nucleus possibly suggesting a malignant cell. Awareness that megakaryocytes may be present within the pulmonary circulation and the observation that this is a single cell within an alveolar capillary should lead to the correct interpretation.

Chapter II
Primary Cancers of the Lung

INTRODUCTION

The great majority of primary lung cancers can be classified into one of the four basic types of carcinomas: adenocarcinoma, squamous cell carcinoma, large cell carcinoma, and small cell carcinoma. Variants of the major cell types are recognized by the World Health Organization, particularly for adenocarcinoma and large cell carcinoma, and there are a number of less common cell types of lung carcinoma. Sarcomas and other types of neoplasm are distinctly rare as primary cancers of the lung. The major differentials for the primary cancers of the lung are metastatic cancers (described in Chapter III) and occasionally differentiation from benign proliferations (discussed in Chapter I).

As noted in Chapter I, a diagnosis of lung carcinoma is often obtained prior to surgical resection by endobronchial biopsy, transbronchial biopsy, or transthoracic needle biopsy, depending on location of the tumor. However, occasionally a definitive diagnosis has not been obtained prior to surgery for technical, logistical, or other reasons and the surgeon may request a frozen section diagnosis at the time of the planned resection. Besides confirming whether or not the patient has malignancy, as discussed in Chapter I, the surgeon may need to know the cell type of the cancer as a basis for proceeding or not proceeding with resection and/or to provide the patient, family, and oncologist some preliminary information about expected prognosis and follow-up care.

SMALL CELL CARCINOMA VERSUS NON-SMALL CELL CARCINOMA

Adenocarcinomas, squamous cell carcinomas, and large cell carcinomas are collectively referred to as non-small cell carcinomas. Currently in most institutions, small cell carcinoma is seldom resected but is treated primarily with chemotherapy and radiation therapy. In contrast, non-small cell carcinomas are treated initially

T.C. Allen, P.T. Cagle, *Frozen Section Library: Lung*,
Frozen Section Library 1, DOI 10.1007/978-0-387-09573-8_2,
© Springer Science+Business Media, LLC 2009

with resection, depending obviously on the stage of disease and other factors. Differentiation of small cell carcinoma from non-small cell carcinoma is therefore a major reason for obtaining frozen section diagnosis of a primary lung cancer when a conclusive preoperative diagnosis has not been obtained.

Pathologists most often encounter small cell carcinomas on small endobronchial or transbronchial biopsies where biopsy artifact, including crush artifact, and "poor preservation" of cells produce characteristic findings of small cell carcinoma: small cells with dense (hyperchromatic) chromatin, absent nucleoli, scant cytoplasm, and often prominent crush artifact. The "better preserved" state of small cell carcinomas seen on frozen section may cause some confusion for the pathologist: the cells may be larger with moderately more abundant cytoplasm, presence of nucleoli, and a more organoid appearance without crush artifact. Individual cells may be very large, although with a very high nucleus-to-cytoplasm ratio. Some variants of non-small cell carcinomas such as basaloid carcinoma may exhibit small cells with very high nucleus-to-cytoplasm ratios that may be confused with small cell carcinoma. Histologic features that differentiate small cell carcinoma from non-small cell carcinomas are listed in Table 2.1.

TABLE 2.1. Histologic features of small cell carcinoma versus non-small cell carcinoma (Figs. 2.1 through 2.11)

Small cell carcinoma	Non-small cell carcinoma
Typically relatively small cells (3–4 times the size of a lymphocyte), but may be larger with variations in size and occasional very large cells	Generally cells are conspicuously larger than cells of small cell carcinoma, but cells may be relatively small in some cell-type variants
Oval to spindle cells consisting primarily of nucleus with scant cytoplasm; better preserved may show more cytoplasm	Typically polygonal or cuboidal cells with moderate-to-abundant cytoplasm depending on specific cell type
Characteristic dense (hyperchromatic), stippled or granular ("salt and pepper") nuclear chromatin	Often open, vesicular nuclei with clumped chromatin
Absent or inconspicuous nucleoli; better preserved may have nucleoli (generally small)	Nucleoli are often present and may be prominent, enlarged and/or multiple

TABLE 2.1. *Continued*

Small cell carcinoma	Non-small cell carcinoma
Molding of cells (nuclei) like pieces of a puzzle; variable organoid growth pattern consistent with a neuroendocrine carcinoma; may have rosettes (should not be confused with glands) or nests with peripheral palisading	Depending on cell type and grade, may have true glands (adenocarcinoma), squamous appearance including keratinization (squamous cell carcinoma), sheets, or nests of cells (all three categories of non-small cell carcinomas)

SMALL CELL CARCINOMA VERSUS LYMPHOMA

Both small cell carcinoma and some types of lymphoma consist of small, round "blue" cells and may involve mediastinal or peribronchial lymph nodes or lung tissue. Generally, proper handling of a lymphoma specimen involves triage of tissue for special studies such as flow cytometric studies. Therefore, differentiation of small cell carcinoma from lymphoma may be an issue at the time of intraoperative consultation for a lung or mediastinal tumor. Lymphomas composed of low-grade small B cells, including some bronchial-associated lymphoid tissue lymphomas, and early peripheral T-cell lymphomas are composed of small lymphocytes with scant cytoplasm that are more likely to cause confusion with small cell carcinoma than are higher-grade large B-cell lymphomas that consist of cells with open, vesicular nuclei, prominent nucleoli, and relatively abundant cytoplasm. Hodgkin lymphomas may exhibit a mixed infiltrate, Hodgkin cells and Reed–Sternberg cells that differentiate it from small cell carcinoma. Histologic features distinguishing small cell carcinoma from lymphomas composed of small lymphocytes are provided in Table 2.2.

CELL TYPES OF NEUROENDOCRINE CARCINOMAS

The neuroendocrine carcinomas of the lung range from indolent typical carcinoid tumors to more aggressive atypical carcinoid tumors to highly aggressive small cell carcinomas and large cell neuroendocrine carcinomas (LCNECs). All of these tumors potentially share some neuroendocrine histologic features such as organoid patterns. Since the majority of carcinoid tumors are cured by resection, and the other neuroendocrine carcinomas may require more extensive surgery or non-surgical therapy, diagnosis of

TABLE 2.2. Histologic features of small cell carcinoma versus lymphoma (Figs. 2.12 through 2.14)

Small cell carcinoma	Lymphoma composed of small lymphocytes
Cohesive cells in clusters, nests, or organoid patterns often with molding of cells (nuclei) like pieces of a puzzle	Discohesive cells in sheets: Depending on cell type, may be arranged in nodular (follicular) pattern
Oval-to-spindle cells consisting primarily of nucleus with scant cytoplasm; better preserved may show more cytoplasm	Depending on cell type, cells may have cerebriform, convoluted nuclei, or angulated or cleaved nuclei, or clumped chromatin; may be mixed with larger cells with vesicular nuclei, distinct nucleoli, and relatively abundant cytoplasm
Characteristic dense (hyperchromatic), stippled or granular ("salt and pepper") nuclear chromatin	
Absent or inconspicuous nucleoli; better preserved may have nucleoli (generally small)	Nucleus may be dense or hyperchromatic with features noted above and may be mixed with larger cells with vesicular nuclei
	Nucleoli may be small, inconspicuous; may be mixed with cells with large and prominent nucleoli

the type of neuroendocrine carcinoma at frozen section may occasionally influence extent of surgical resection and provides information about expected prognosis and probable follow-up care that the surgeon may wish to convey to the patient, family, or oncologist postoperatively. Histologic features that separate the different categories of neuroendocrine carcinomas are given in Table 2.3.

BRONCHIOLOALVEOLAR CARCINOMAS

By current definition, bronchioloalveolar carcinomas (BACs) are in-situ carcinomas and, therefore, are presumed "cured" by surgical resection. Although the definitive diagnosis of BAC requires examination of the complete specimen for areas of invasion, the information that a tumor may be potentially cured by resection may be useful knowledge at the time of intraoperative consultation. Features of BAC are given in Table 2.4.

TABLE 2.3. Histologic features of pulmonary neuroendocrine carcinomas (Figs. 2.15 through 2.18)

Typical carcinoid tumor	Atypical carcinoid tumor	Small cell carcinoma	Large cell neuroendocrine carcinoma
Classic growth patterns of carcinoid tumor include organoid and trabecular patterns	Atypical carcinoid tumors show histologic features similar to typical carcinoid tumors but with additional findings of necrosis and more than two mitoses per high-power field.	Small cell carcinomas have small cell size, approximately 3–4 times the size of a resting lymphocyte	Neuroendocrine morphology, typically consisting of an organoid or nested pattern, must be present
■ Unusual growth patterns include papillary, pseudoglandular, follicular, prominent rosettes, and spindle cell pattern is often present in the same tumor	■ Necrosis is typically present centrally within organoid nests and may be punctate; zones of "infarct-like" necrosis may occur	■ Cells have scant cytoplasm, granular chromatin, oval-to-spindle cell shape, absent or inconspicuous nucleoli, and typically prominent necrosis	■ Peripheral palisading around tumor nests is common, and rosette formation may be prominent
■ Carcinoid cells generally have uniform, round nuclei with finely granular chromatin, inconspicuous nucleoli, and scant-to-moderately abundant eosinophilic cytoplasm	■ Mitotic activity should be assessed in the most active areas; ideally, three sets of 10 high-power fields should be counted and averaged	■ In larger biopsies or resection specimens, cells may appear better preserved and larger, with more discernible cytoplasm	■ Necrosis may occur centrally within nests
■ Prominent nucleoli may occasionally occur		■ Transbronchial biopsies typically show sheets of cells with prominent crush artifact	■ LCNECs have a mitotic rate greater than 10 per 10 high-power fields, typically averaging 70 per 10 high-power fields
		■ Larger specimens may show a more obvious neuroendocrine growth	■ Features differentiating LCNEC from small cell carcinoma include large cell size, polygonal shape, moderately abundant cytoplasm, coarse or

TABLE 2.3. *Continued*

Typical carcinoid tumor	Atypical carcinoid tumor	Small cell carcinoma	Large cell neuroendocrine carcinoma
■ Carcinoid cells may occasionally show clear cytoplasm, oncocytic cytoplasm, granular basophilic "acinic" cytoplasm, and intracytoplasmic melanin pigment ■ Cellular pleomorphism may be marked, even in typical carcinoid, and is not a criterion for distinguishing typical carcinoid from atypical carcinoid ■ Stroma is typically delicate and highly vascular; however, dense hyaline collagen, amyloid-like stroma, metaplastic cartilage, or bone may occasionally occur		pattern, including organoid pattern with peripheral palisading, rosettes, and pseudopapillary pattern	vesicular chromatin rather than finely granular chromatin, frequent nucleoli, and lack of prominent spindle morphology ■ LCNEC may occur combined with conventional adenocarcinoma, squamous carcinoma, or carcinoma with spindle cell features.

TABLE 2.4. Features of BAC (Figs. 2.19 through 2.26)

- Uniformly atypical cells grow in continuous row over intact alveolar septa (lepidic pattern)
- No invasion of interstitium although there may be alveolar collapse with "entrapped" spaces lined by BAC that resembles invasion (invasion usually associated with small acini, cribriform or angulated glands, or individual cells within stroma)
- Cells generally columnar, but may occasionally be cuboidal
- Nuclear stratification and tufting may be present
- Papillary structures may be present

NON-SMALL CELL CARCINOMAS

Further subclassification of a non-small cell carcinoma as an adenocarcinoma, squamous cell carcinoma, or large cell carcinoma may be possible at the time of frozen section, but is typically not mandatory. Lung cancers are sometimes heterogeneous, and frozen section sampling may not include all cell types that are identified upon wider permanent sectioning. Differentiation of cell types is increasingly important for new therapies such as targeted molecular therapies. However, since these treatments are not going to be instituted immediately at the time of surgery, further differentiation of cell type can await permanent sections.

TABLE 2.5. Features of Atypical Adenomatous Hyperplasia (Fig. 2.27)

- Cells with mild atypia growing along intact alveolar septa in a "hobnail" or "picket-fence" pattern
- Sharp demarcation from adjacent lung parenchyma
- No condition in background to cause pneumocyte hyperplasia
- Usually less than 5 mm but may be larger
- May be difficult to differentiate from bronchioloalveolar carcinoma
- Lesions < 5 mm with significant cytologic atypia may be small bronchioloalveolar carcinomas

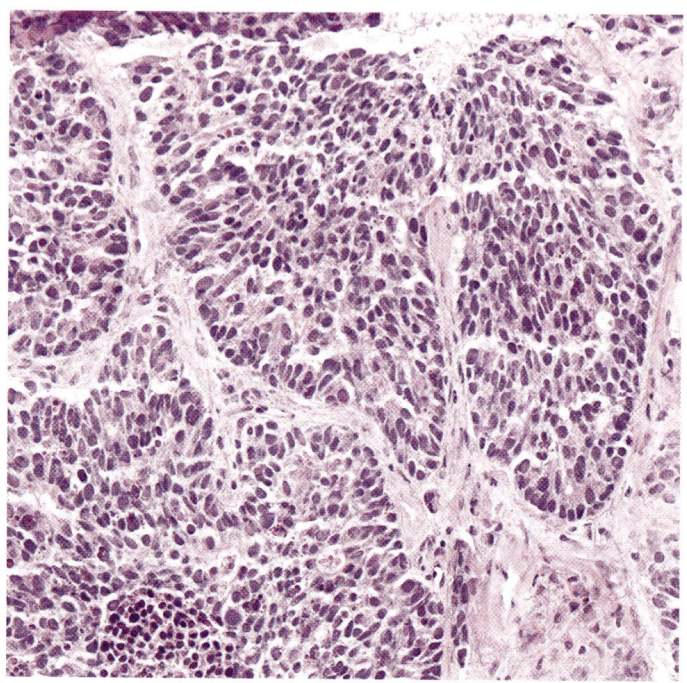

FIGURE 2.1. Medium-power view shows frozen section of a small cell carcinoma composed of nests of cells with scant cytoplasm. The cells are arranged in an organoid pattern with pseudorosettes and peripheral palisading. There is focal tumor necrosis. Compared to the appearance of small cell carcinoma on transbronchial biopsy, the carcinoma cells show some variability in size and focally more cytoplasm on frozen section.

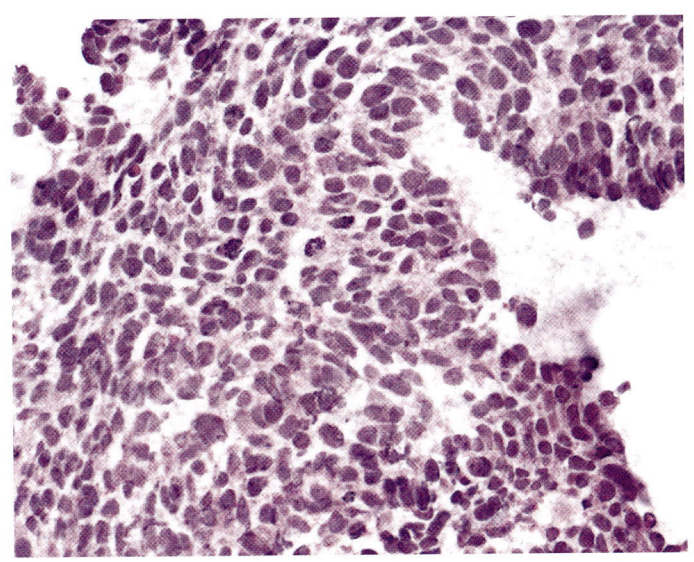

FIGURE 2.2. High-power view shows classic features of small cell carcinoma on frozen section: nests of cohesive oval-to-rounded cells with relatively scant cytoplasm, smudged dark nuclear chromatin, and nuclear molding. In contrast to the typical appearance on transbronchial biopsy, crush artifact is not noted and some of the cells show nucleoli.

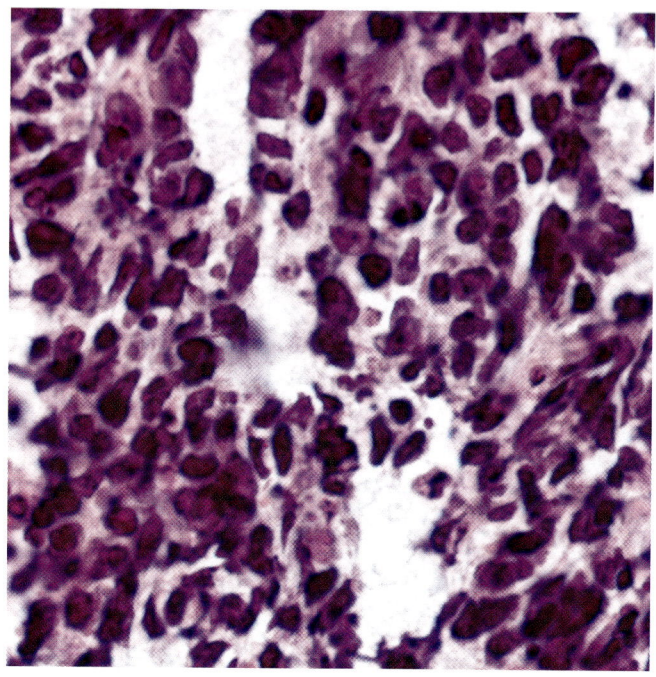

FIGURE 2.3. High-power view shows some cells with angulated-to-spindle shaped, dark nuclei with relatively scant cytoplasm characteristic of small cell carcinoma on frozen section.

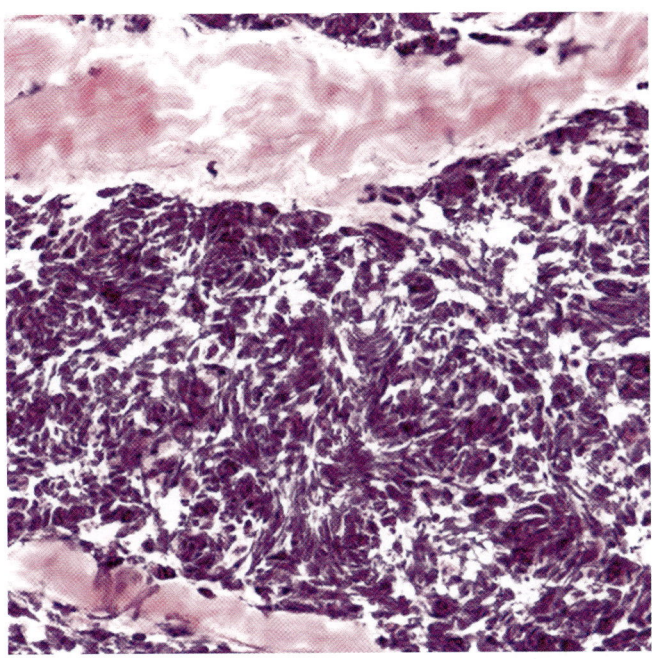

FIGURE 2.4. A spindle appearance of the cells is emphasized in this medium-power view of a frozen section of small cell carcinoma.

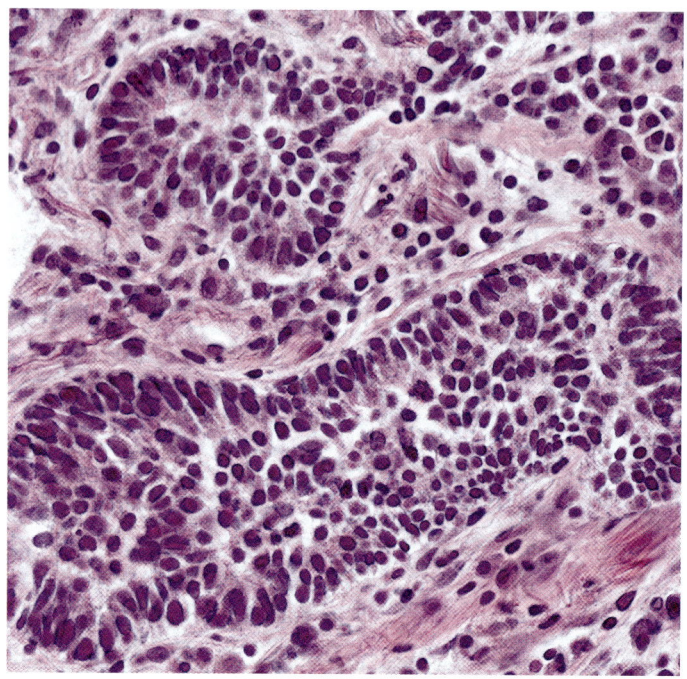

FIGURE 2.5. These nests of small cell carcinoma have prominent peripheral palisading on frozen section.

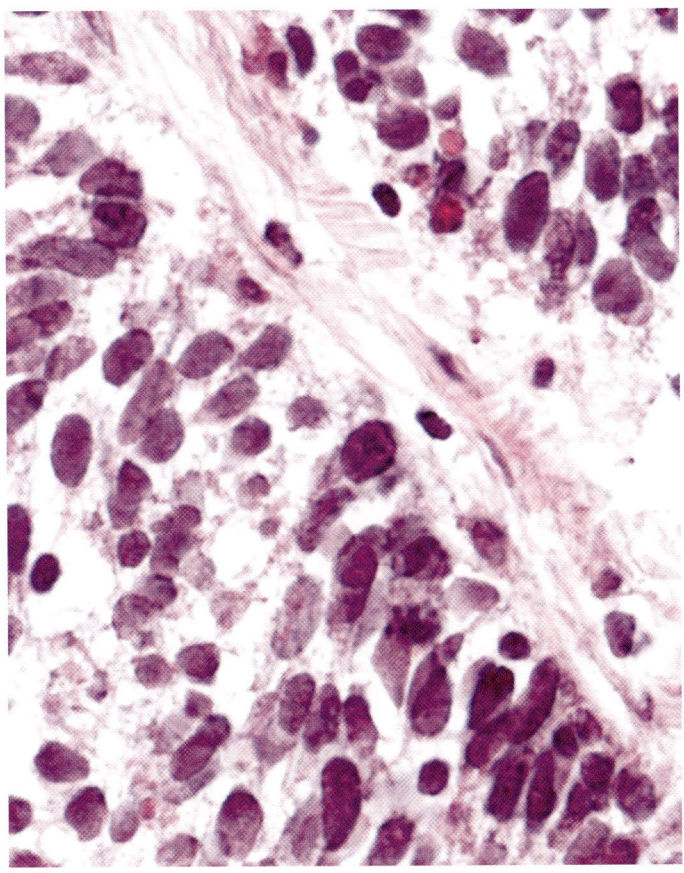

FIGURE 2.6. The size of the small cell carcinoma cells is more than twice the size of the lymphocytes in the same field. On this frozen section, nucleoli can be observed in some of the carcinoma cells.

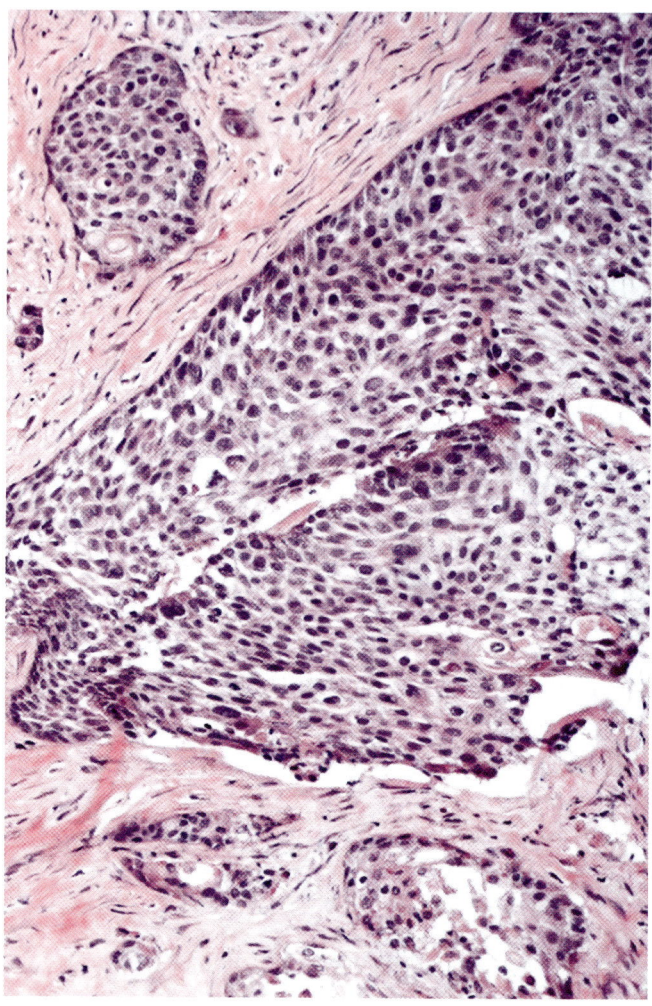

FIGURE 2.7. In contrast to small cell carcinoma, this frozen section of a non-small cell carcinoma shows nests of cohesive epithelial cells with comparatively abundant cytoplasm.

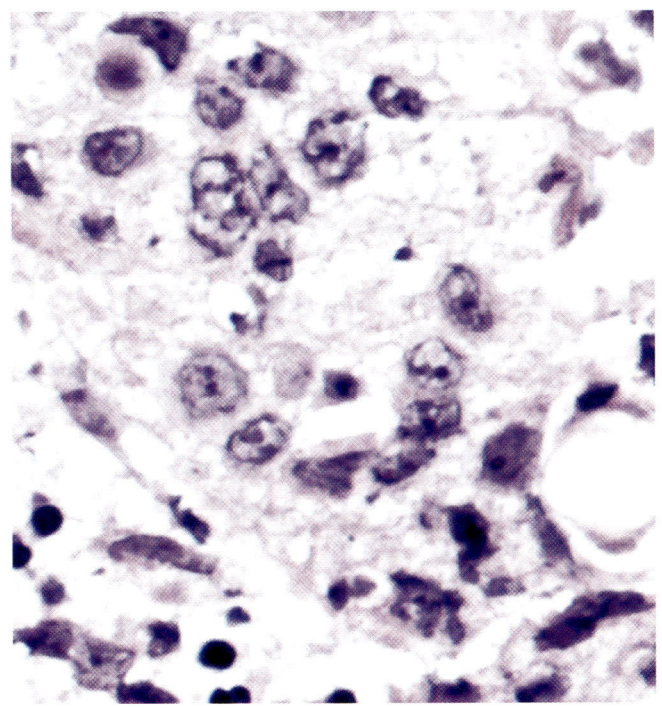

FIGURE 2.8. High-power view of a frozen section of a non-small cell carcinoma shows polygonal cells with relatively abundant cytoplasm, open vesicular nuclei, and conspicuous nucleoli.

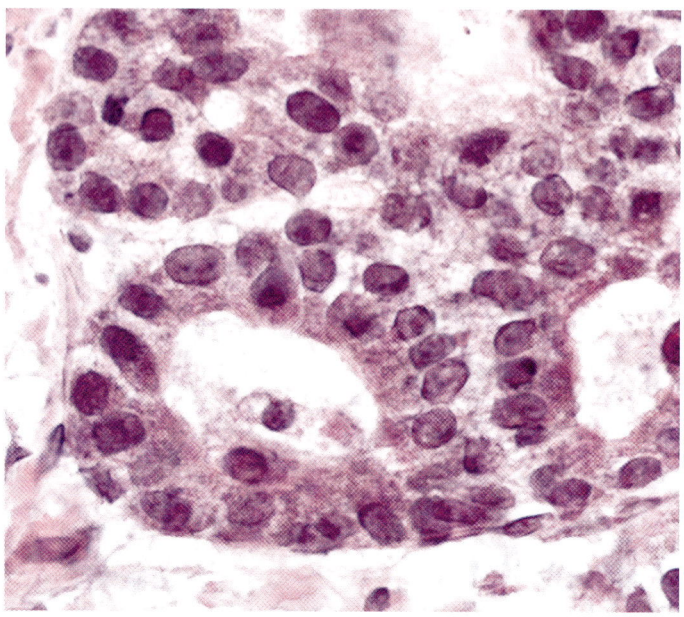

FIGURE 2.9. High-power view of frozen section of an adenocarcinoma shows glands lined by cells with relatively abundant cytoplasm and nuclei with prominent nucleoli.

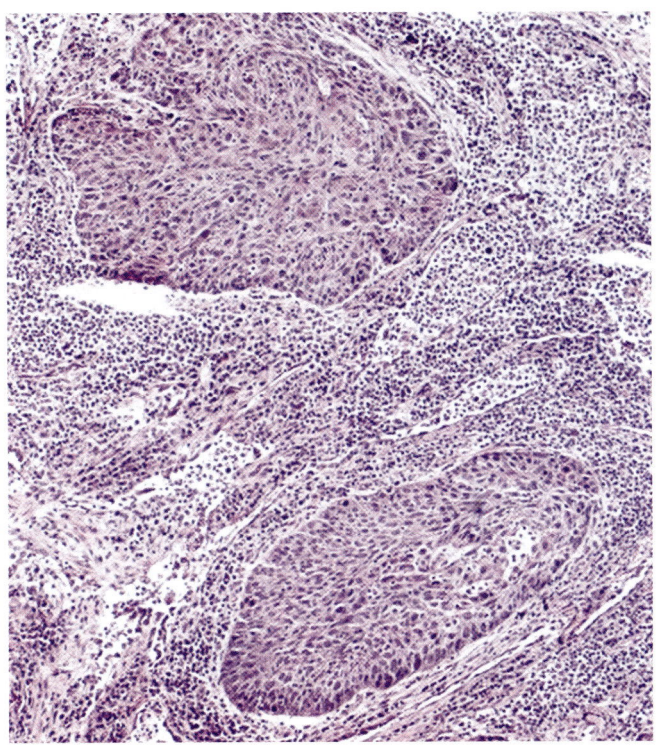

FIGURE 2.10. At low power on frozen section, nests of non-small cell carcinoma may superficially resemble small cell carcinoma when the amount of cytoplasm is relatively less than the typical non-small cell carcinoma. Closer examination of the cytologic features under higher power should permit correct diagnosis.

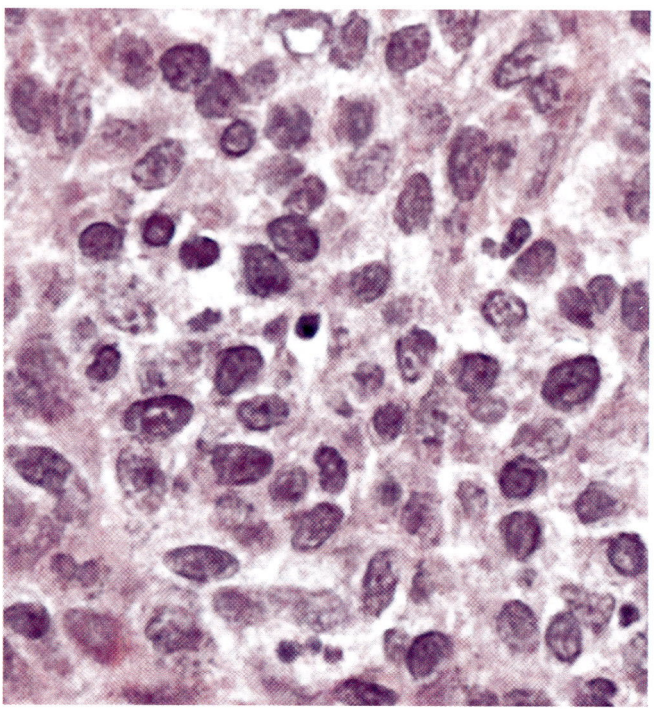

FIGURE 2.11. High-power view of cancer in Fig. 2.10 shows that the cells consistently have more cytoplasm than small cell carcinoma, although less than the classic non-small carcinoma. Most importantly, the nuclei consistently have an open chromatin with prominent nucleoli as compared to small cell carcinoma. Although small cell carcinoma on frozen section may have nucleoli and relatively more cytoplasm than on transbronchial biopsy, the overall cytologic features should allow one to distinguish a small cell carcinoma from a non-small cell carcinoma.

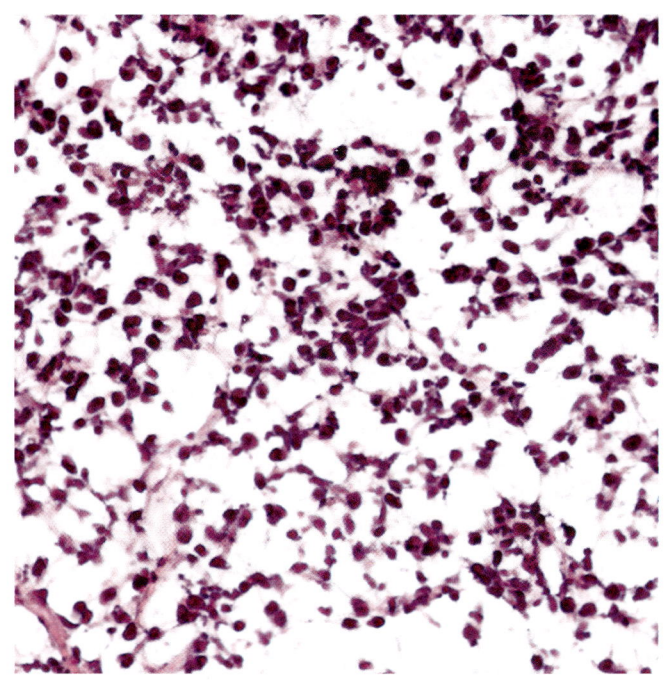

FIGURE 2.12. This touch preparation of a lung mass performed at the time of intraoperative consultation shows discohesive round cells with scanty cytoplasm. The lack of cohesion and the other cytologic features of lymphoid cells allow one to make a diagnosis of lymphoma.

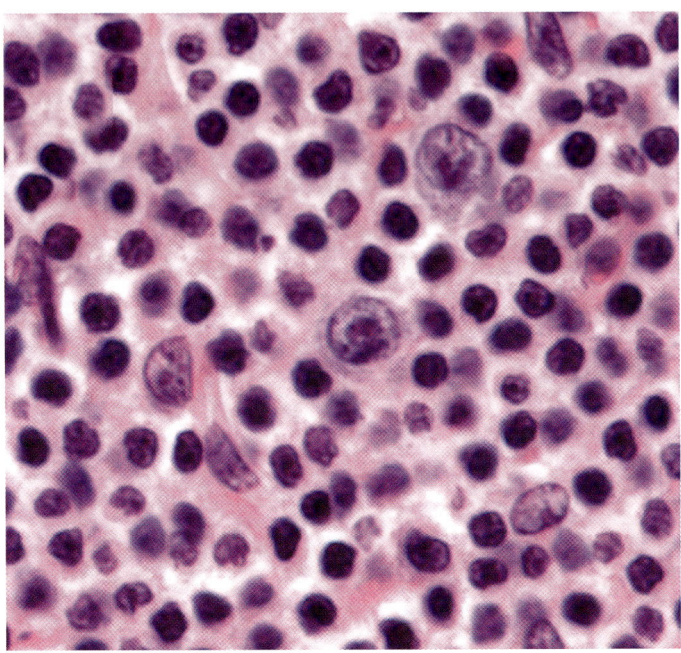

FIGURE 2.13. This frozen section of a low-grade B-cell lymphoma of the bronchial-associated lymphoid tissue shows small lymphoid cells that can be distinguished from small cell carcinoma by their relatively uniform round shape and lack of cohesion and molding. In addition, there are interspersed larger cells with vesicular nuclei, prominent nucleoli, and comparatively abundant cytoplasm, features that are not expected with small cell carcinoma.

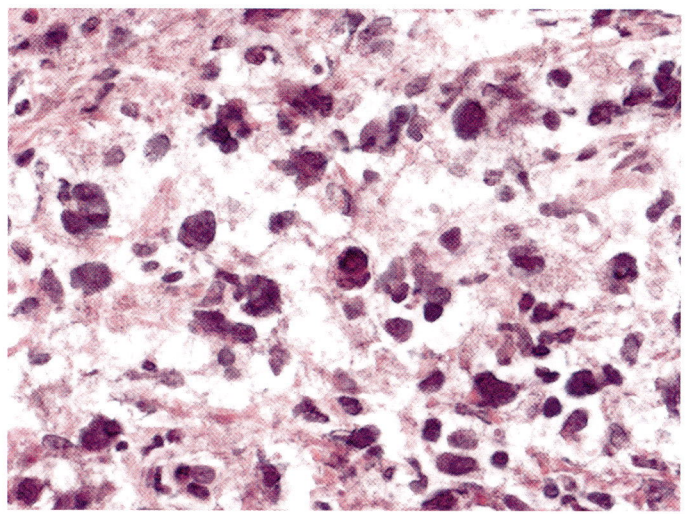

FIGURE 2.14. Lymphocyte-depleted Hodgkin lymphoma of the lung shows cells with prominent nucleoli on this frozen section. The scattered cytologically atypical cells suggest a diagnosis other than small cell or non-small cell carcinoma by their lack of cohesive nests of cells. Other types of Hodgkin lymphoma may exhibit a mixed inflammatory background. However, primary Hodgkin lymphoma of the lung is rare and, in the absence of clinical history, it may be necessary to defer diagnosis until permanent sections are available.

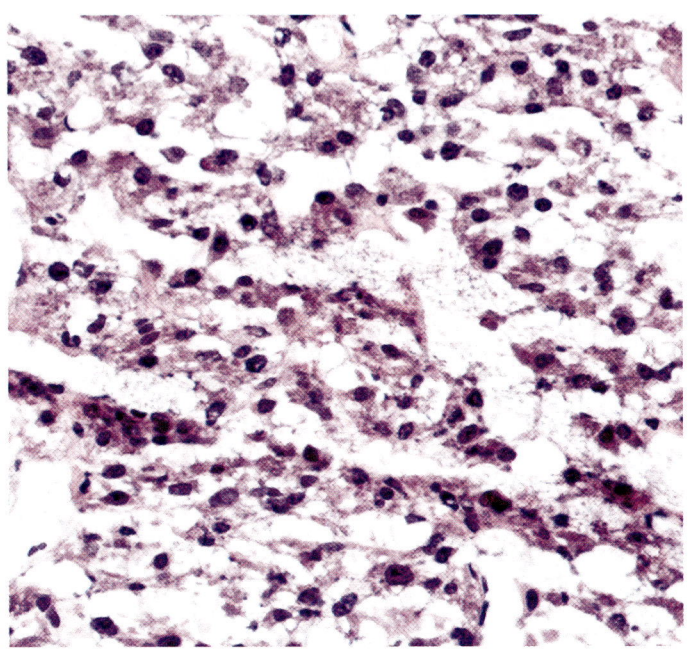

FIGURE 2.15. On frozen section, this carcinoid tumor consists of plasmacytoid-like cells arranged in a vaguely organoid pattern. The nuclei are relatively round and the cells have comparatively abundant cytoplasm. Frozen section artifact slightly distorts the classic features of a carcinoid tumor but if analyzed objectively, the features are present.

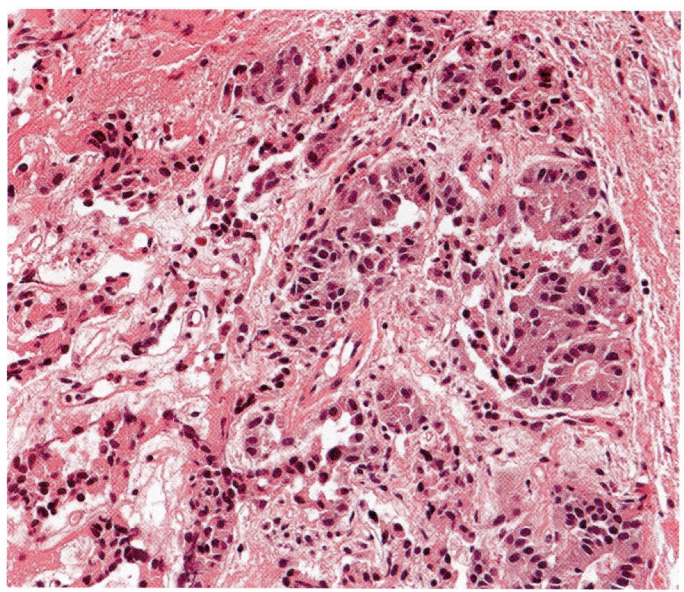

FIGURE 2.16. This carcinoid tumor consists of relatively uniform cells with comparatively bland nuclei and abundant oncocytic cytoplasm arranged in an organoid pattern. There is some distortion of features due to frozen section artifact and procedural artifact and the tumor has been sampled near its margin providing a more infiltrative appearance rather than nests of cells. The differential diagnosis in this case might include adenocarcinoma rather than small cell carcinoma due to the presence of the "gland-like" structures and abundant eosinophilic cytoplasm. However, the nuclei are too regular and proportionately too small relative to the cytoplasm for this to be an adenocarcinoma.

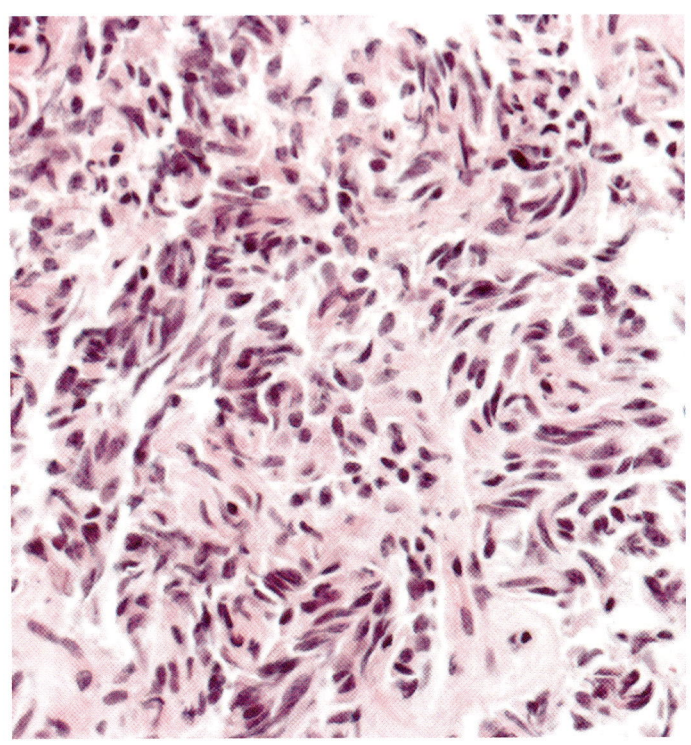

FIGURE 2.17. This carcinoid tumor is composed of spindle cells and on frozen section other spindle cell neoplasms may enter into the differential diagnosis. Clues to the correct diagnosis include an organoid pattern at low power and areas of characteristic carcinoid tumor.

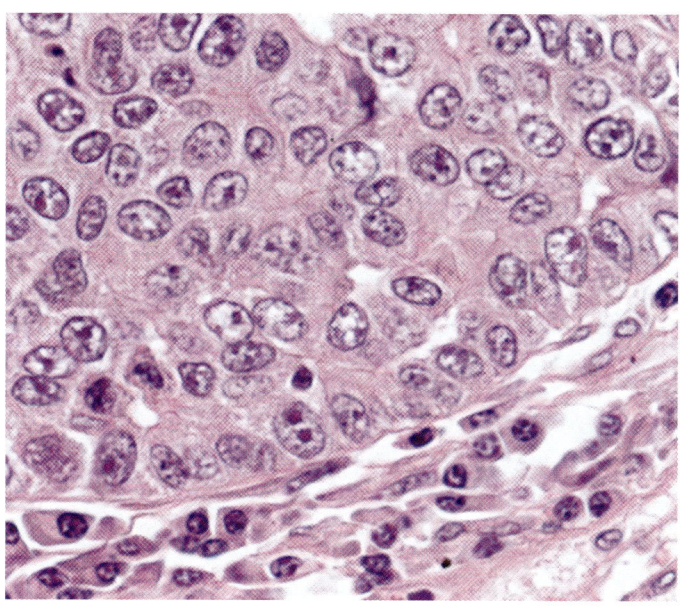

Figure 2.18. On frozen section, this large cell neuroendocrine carcinoma (LCNEC) is composed of cells with open vesicular nuclei, prominent nucleoli, and ample cytoplasm. The size of these cells can be compared to the size of the adjacent lymphocytes and plasma cells. Obviously, based on the cytology of the tumor cells, other categories of non-small cell carcinoma, for example adenocarcinoma, enter into the differential diagnosis for LCNEC. The diagnosis of a neuroendocrine carcinoma is based on the low-power organoid pattern and confirmed by immunopositivity for neuroendocrine markers on the permanent sections.

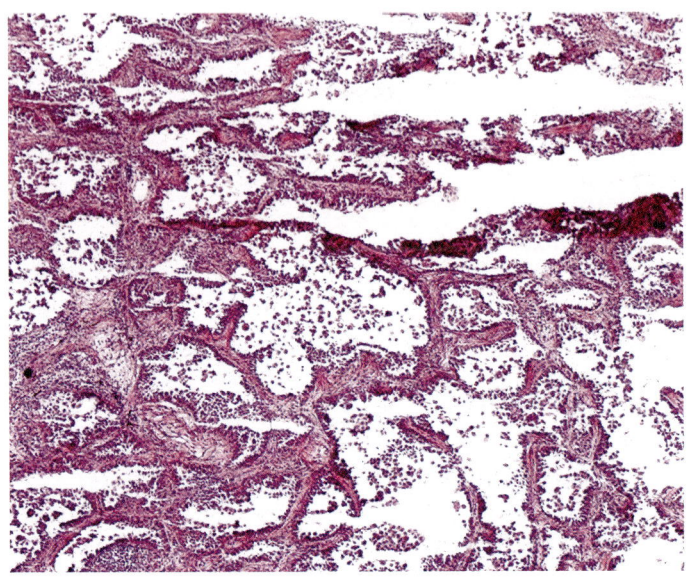

FIGURE 2.19. Low-power view of a BAC frozen section shows intact alveolar septa lined by relatively uniform malignant columnar cells. No definite invasion into the underlying stroma is identified.

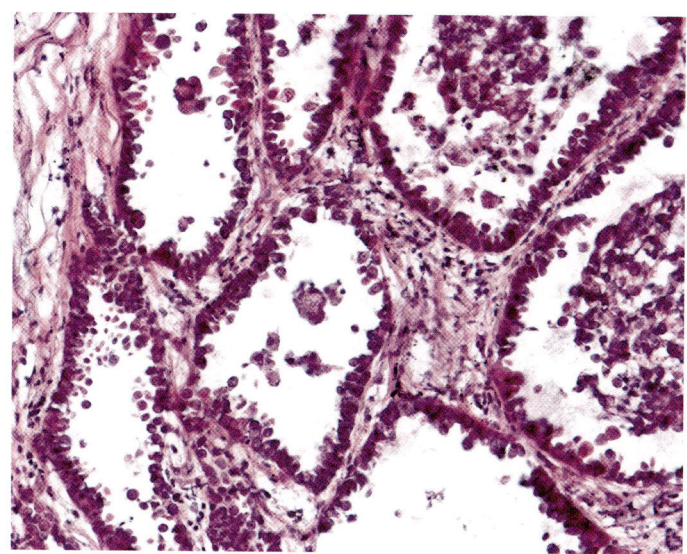

FIGURE 2.20. High-power view of frozen section shows relatively uniform malignant columnar cells of BAC lining intact alveolar septa with no invasion into the stroma identified.

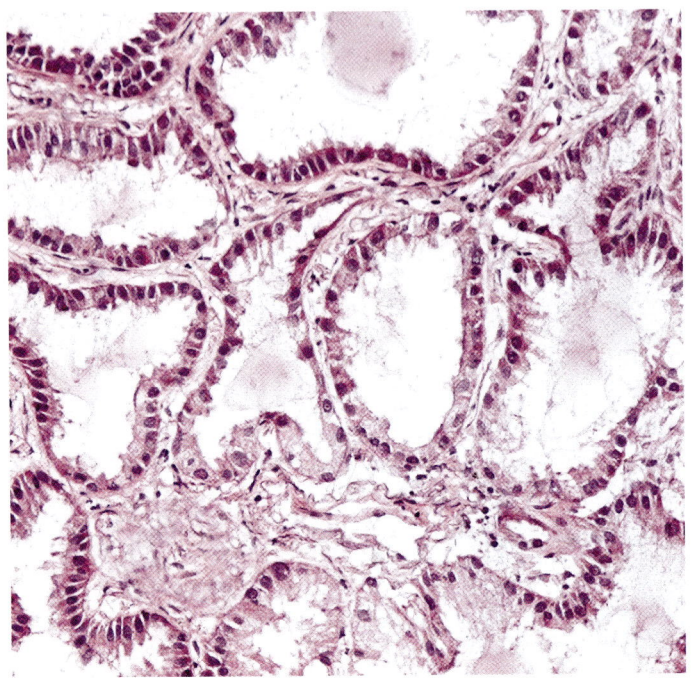

FIGURE 2.21. Frozen section high-power view of a different BAC demonstrates similar features to the cancer in Fig. 2.19. This tumor also has fairly uniform columnar cells growing in a lepidic pattern over thickened alveolar septa without invasion.

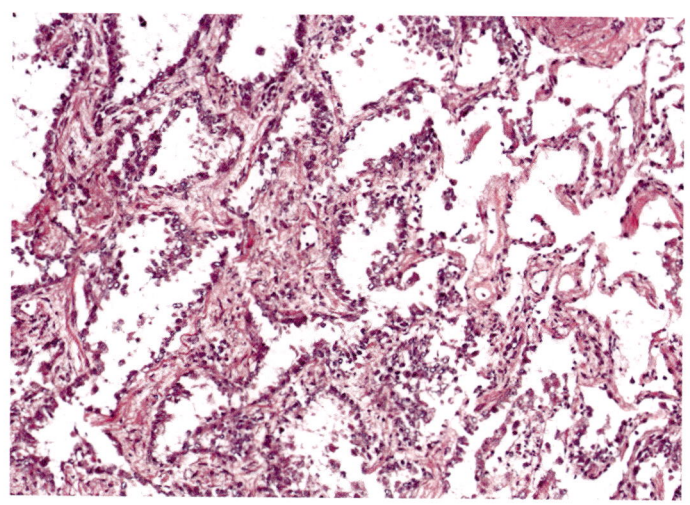

FIGURE 2.22. Another feature of BAC that may be seen on frozen section if the margin of the tumor is sampled. The growth of the malignant columnar cells along thickened alveolar septa is sharply demarcated from the adjacent uninvolved alveolar septa which are of normal thickness and not lined by atypical cells. In contrast, the margin of a reactive proliferation tends to blend atypical, less atypical, and normal cells rather than demonstrate a sharp boundary between atypical and normal cells. Atypical adenomatous hyperplasia also enters into the differential diagnosis of reactive atypia and BAC and is illustrated in Fig. 2.27.

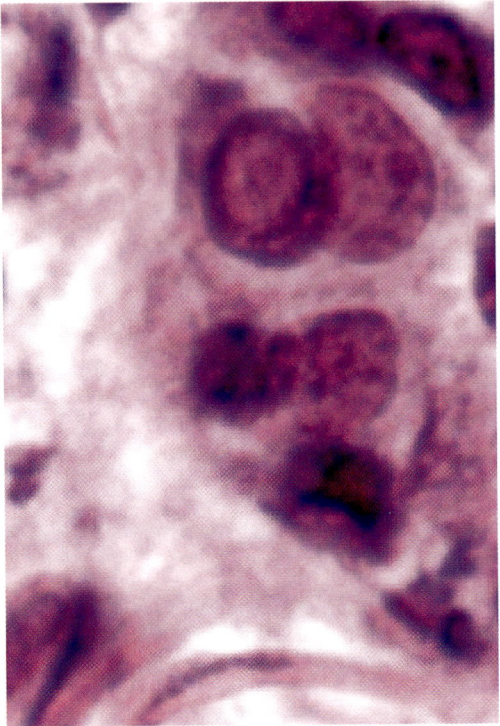

FIGURE 2.23. Intranuclear inclusions, illustrated in this frozen section of a BAC, may be numerous and large in BACs as compared to the occasional smaller intranuclear inclusions that may be seen in reactive alveolar epithelium.

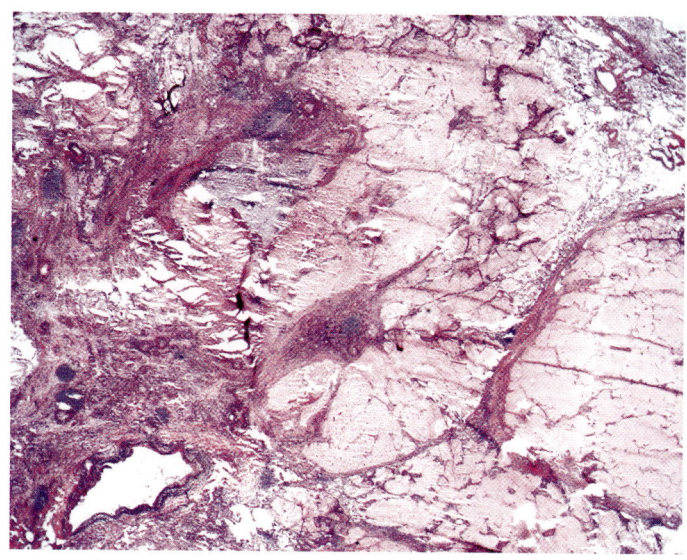

FIGURE 2.24. Low-power view of frozen section of mucinous BAC shows mucin-filled alveolar spaces. No nests or sheets of tumor cells are observed.

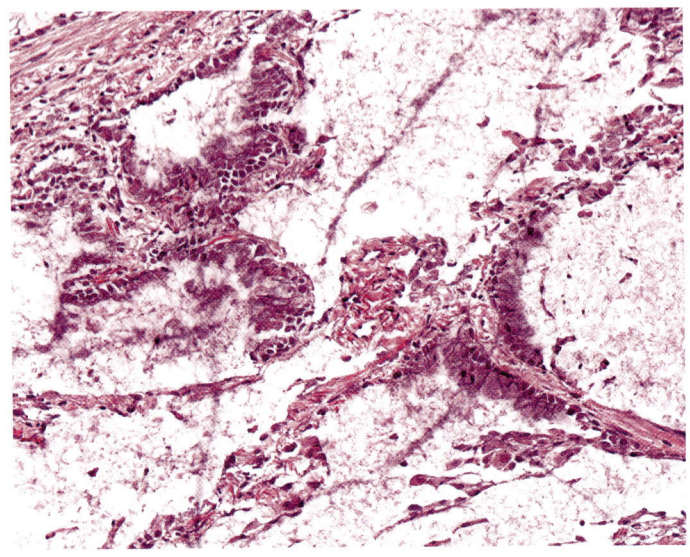

FIGURE 2.25. Medium-power view shows that some alveolar septa are partially lined by relatively uniform goblet cells consistent with a mucinous BAC.

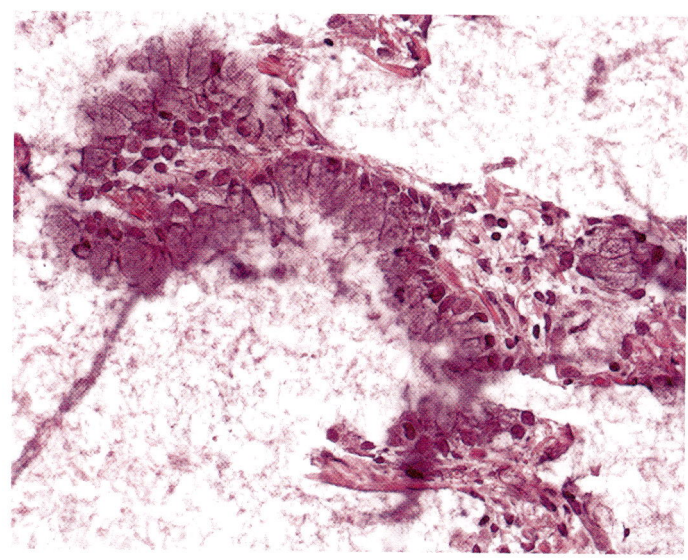

FIGURE 2.26. High-power view shows row of uniform goblet cells with bland nuclei lining an alveolar septum consistent with a mucinous BAC.

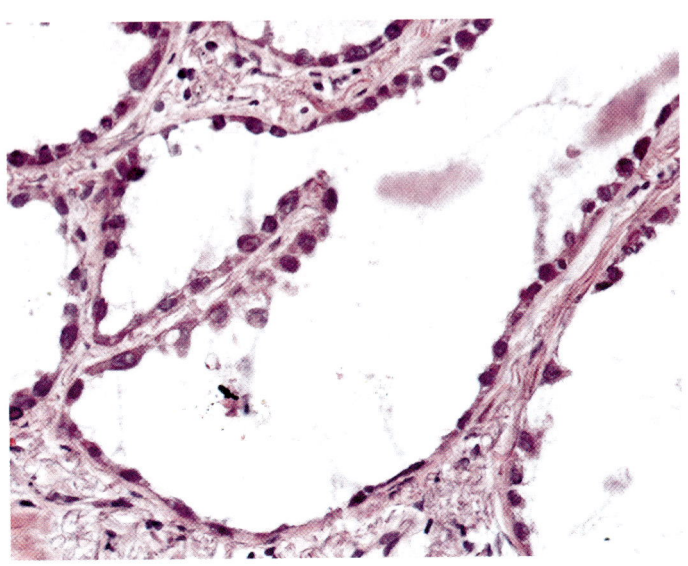

FIGURE 2.27. High-power view of atypical adenomatous hyperplasia from a frozen section consists of cuboidal cells with mild cytologic atypia growing in a picket fence pattern along intact alveolar septa. Atypical adenomatous hyperplasia may occur at the margin of a peripheral adenocarcinoma or as a small incidental lesion in lung tissue resected for a lung cancer or other reason. The latter is more likely to raise concerns about a primary or metastatic BAC. Features characteristic of atypical adenomatous hyperplasia are listed in Table 2.5.

Chapter III
Metastases to the Lung

INTRODUCTION

Cancers from virtually every site in the body can metastasize to the lung. In most cases, the site of the primary cancer is already known, appropriate chemotherapy or other modalities are instituted, and surgical resection of lung metastases is not performed. Surgical biopsy or excision of a metastasis may be performed to rule out a second primary cancer arising in the lung or for treatment of a solitary or limited number of metastases in the lung. Occasionally, the surgical biopsy may be performed to determine the primary site of a cancer of unknown origin: is the lung mass a primary lung tumor or from another site and, if the latter, where? Due to more sophisticated imaging techniques than in the past, this latter reason for sampling a metastatic tumor is less frequent than previously, but still occurs occasionally.

A frozen section may be requested for a metastatic tumor to determine if the tumor is a likely metastasis, and hence no lobectomy or pneumonectomy is warranted, or a lung primary which may require additional surgery for staging and a more extensive definitive procedure such as a lobectomy. If a metastasis is already the working diagnosis, a frozen section may be used to confirm that diagnostic tissue has been obtained or that a solitary metastasis was successfully excised. Occasionally, the histology of the tumor at frozen section of a suspected lung primary may raise suspicions that the tumor is not a lung primary after all. Communication with the surgeon is essential to determine if another primary site is already known and to decide whether more extensive surgery is justified.

Immunohistochemistry and molecular techniques to confirm the primary site of a metastasis cannot be performed at the time of frozen section. However, the histologic features of the tumor may be helpful in suggesting the likely primary site and can be discussed with the surgeon. In some cases, the histologic features of lung cancer and cancer from one or more other primary sites may overlap.

T.C. Allen, P.T. Cagle, *Frozen Section Library: Lung*,
Frozen Section Library 1, DOI 10.1007/978-0-387-09573-8_3,
© Springer Science+Business Media, LLC 2009

Although final diagnosis may have to await permanent sections including special studies such as immunostains, the pathologist can convey the differential diagnosis to the surgeon so that a fully informed clinical decision can be made. Some of the specific scenarios that the pathologist may encounter with metastatic cancers are discussed below.

HISTOPATHOLOGIC FEATURES FAVORING PRIMARY LUNG CARCINOMA

Histopathologic features that may favor a primary lung carcinoma at frozen section are listed in Table 3.1. These features are typical of primary lung carcinomas, but are not observed in all cases and their presence depends on the cell type, location of the tumor, type of specimen, and other factors. Therefore, if one or more of these features is present, they support a diagnosis of primary lung carcinoma, but their absence does not, by itself, exclude a primary lung carcinoma.

HISTOPATHOLOGIC FEATURES FAVORING METASTATIC CANCER

If the surgeon has not provided information that the patient has a known non-pulmonary primary cancer, the pathologist must be suspicious that the histopathologic pattern represents something other than a lung carcinoma in order to suggest the correct diagnosis. The entire spectrum of histopathologic features of non-pulmonary metastases cannot be described here, but some relatively common and well-recognized histopathologic features of metastases are summarized in Table 3.2. The presence of multiple tumor nodules is often cited as evidence of metastases (Fig. 3.1), but it should be noted that

TABLE 3.1. Histopathologic features favoring a primary lung carcinoma at frozen section

---

Primary adenocarcinoma
- Mixed histopathologic patterns including solid, acinar, papillary, and/or bronchioloalveolar (lepidic) architecture
- Often moderately-to-poorly differentiated
- Adjacent atypical adenomatous hyperplasia in parenchyma surrounding peripheral adenocarcinomas
- Central scar may be present

Primary squamous cell carcinoma
- Adjacent squamous metaplasia or dysplasia of airway epithelium
- Typically moderately to poorly differentiated

TABLE 3.2. Histopathologic features of common non-pulmonary metastases at frozen section (Figs. 3.2 through 3.10)

Metastatic adenocarcinoma
- Cribriform pattern suggests colon primary
- "Dirty" necrosis suggests colon primary
- Relatively bland or uniform cells in nests or single file cords suggests breast primary
- Small glands with relatively bland cells suggests prostate primary

Metastatic squamous cell carcinoma
- Well-differentiated keratinizing squamous cell carcinoma suggests head and neck primary

multiple nodules could represent synchronous primary lung carcinomas or lung cancer that has metastasized within the lungs rather than from a non-pulmonary primary. The differential diagnoses of several distinctive histopathologic patterns which may be seen with either primary or metastatic tumors are given in Table 3.3.

TABLE 3.3. Differential diagnosis of distinctive histopathologic patterns (Figs. 3.11 through 3.19)

Primary clear cell tumors of the lung
　　Clear cell adenocarcinoma or clear cell squamous cell carcinoma
　　Clear cell tumor ("Sugar tumor" or PEComa)

Metastatic clear cell tumors
　　Renal cell carcinoma
　　Clear cell carcinoma of the ovary, endometrium, or cervix
　　Clear cell melanoma/clear cell sarcoma of soft parts
　　Adrenal cortical carcinoma
　　Alveolar soft part sarcoma
　　Clear cell diffuse malignant mesothelioma
　　Rare clear cell variants of other cancer types (hepatocellular clear cell variant; clear cell adenocarcinoma of the urinary bladder, etc.)

Primary papillary tumors of the lung
　　Papillary adenocarcinoma
　　Adenocarcinoma with micropapillary component
　　Bronchioloalveolar carcinoma with papillary component
　　Sclerosing hemangioma
　　Pseudopapillary pattern of small cell carcinoma
　　Papilloma/Papillary squamous cell carcinoma

TABLE 3.3. *Continued*

Metastatic papillary tumors
  Papillary thyroid carcinoma
  Papillary renal cell carcinoma
  Papillary serous ovarian carcinoma
  Papillary endometrial carcinoma and endocervical carcinoma
  Papillary urothelial (transitional cell) carcinoma
  Papillary pancreatic adenocarcinoma
  Papillary breast carcinoma
  Papillary cholangiocarcinoma
  Serous papillary adenocarcinoma of the peritoneum
  Tubulopapillary diffuse malignant mesothelioma
Primary small blue cell tumors of the lung
  Small cell carcinoma
  Carcinoid tumor and atypical carcinoid tumor
  Lymphoma
  Carcinoid tumorlets
  Desmoplastic small round cell tumor
  Primitive neuroectodermal tumor (Askin tumor)

Metastatic small blue cell tumors
  Lymphoma
  Lobular breast carcinoma
  Nonpulmonary small cell carcinoma
  Desmoplastic small round cell tumor
  Ewing's sarcoma
  Melanoma
  Rhabdomyosarcoma
  Small cell diffuse malignant mesothelioma

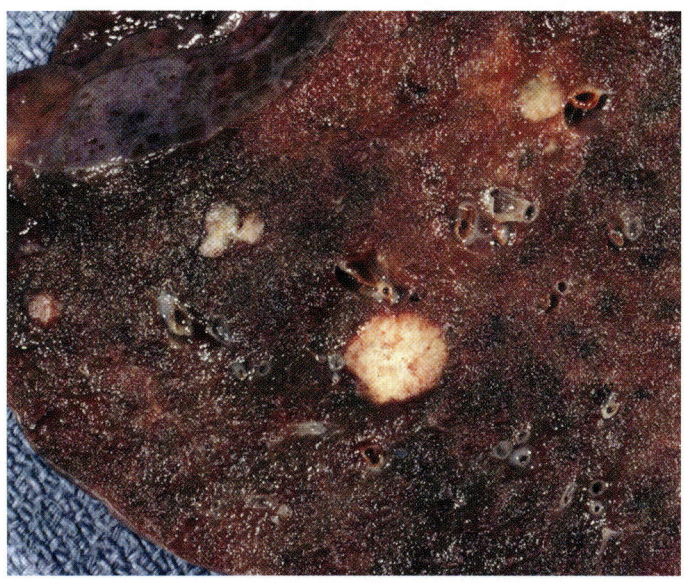

FIGURE 3.1. Gross of cut surface of lung with multiple tan-yellow-to-gray-white nodules of metastatic cancer scattered in the parenchyma. Multiple tumor nodules like this are considered evidence of metastatic cancer. Multiple nodules are not always the result of metastases from distant primary sites. It should be remembered that the lung can sometimes have two or more synchronous primary cancers and that metastases within the lungs from a lung primary can also occur.

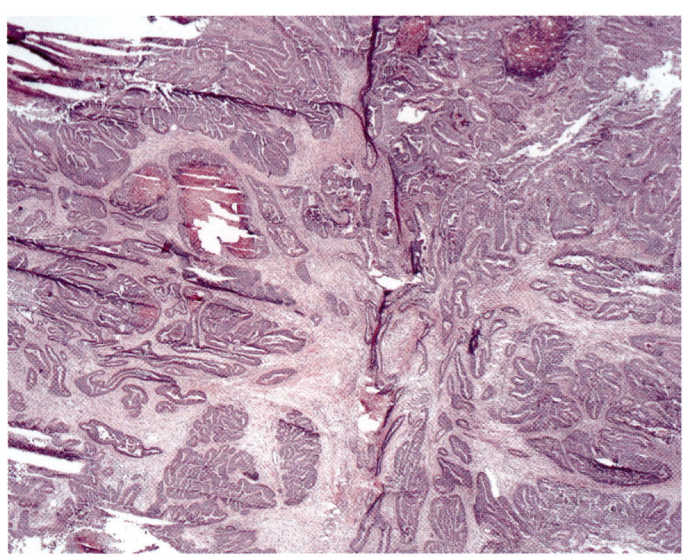

FIGURE 3.2. Low-power view of a metastatic adenocarcinoma of the colon seen in a frozen section of a lung mass shows complex glands embedded in desmoplastic tissue. The glands are arranged in a vaguely whirled fashion around a relatively central focus of desmoplasia. Even at low power, the histopathologic features suggest an adenocarcinoma of the colon including complex, cribriform glands, columnar malignant cells, and "dirty" necrosis. In addition to mild blurring of detail by frozen section artifact, there are some artifactual tears and folding in the tissue.

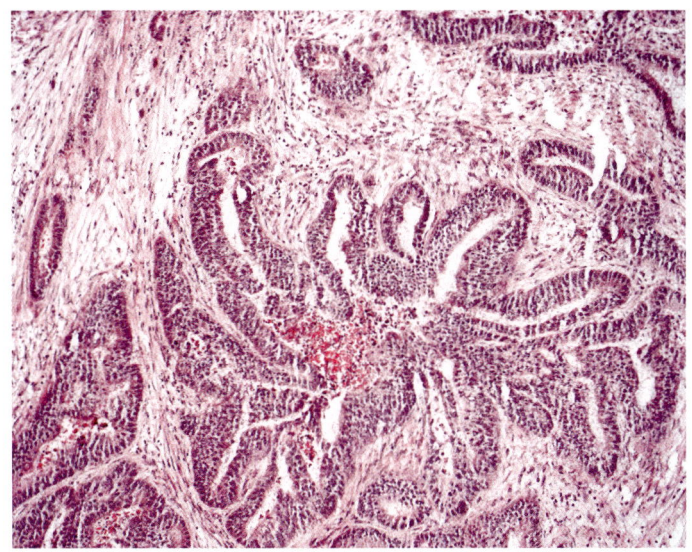

FIGURE 3.3. High-power view of the metastatic adenocarcinoma shows histopathologic features of a primary colon cancer including complicated, cribriforming glands lined by stratified malignant columnar cells and a focus of "dirty" necrosis. Although it is not impossible for a primary lung adenocarcinoma to rarely exhibit these combined features, this histopathologic pattern is highly characteristic of metastatic adenocarcinoma of the colon and should suggest the likelihood of a colon primary in assessing the differential diagnosis. In most cases, it will be known that the patient has a history of a primary colon cancer. If not, immunostains may be helpful later when permanent sections are available.

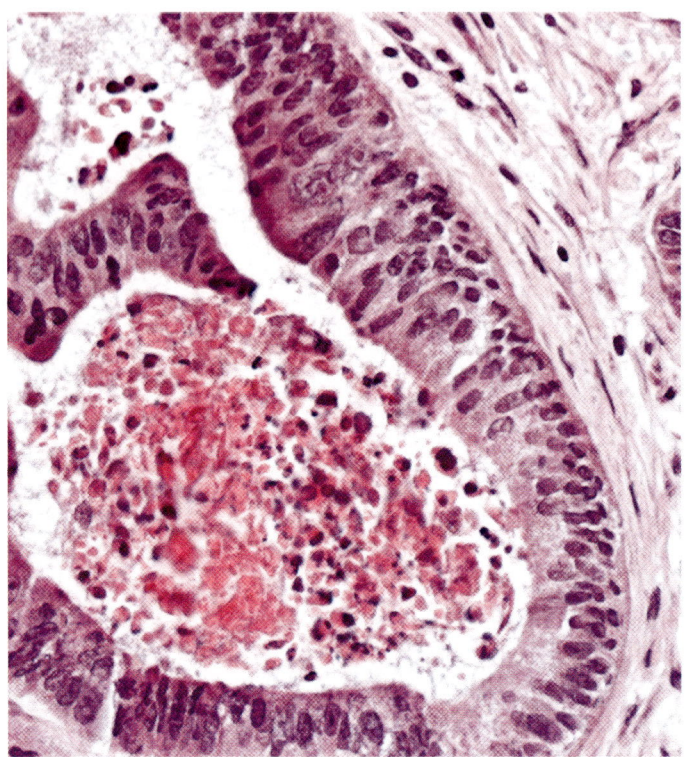

FIGURE 3.4. High-power view highlights "dirty" necrosis within the lumen of a gland lined by stratified malignant columnar cells, some of which exhibit prominent nucleoli. The "dirty" necrosis consists of eosinophilic amorphous necrotic material admixed with hematoxylin-staining nuclear debris and inflammatory cell nuclei. "Dirty" necrosis can be seen in other types of cancer, but is characteristic of colon adenocarcinoma.

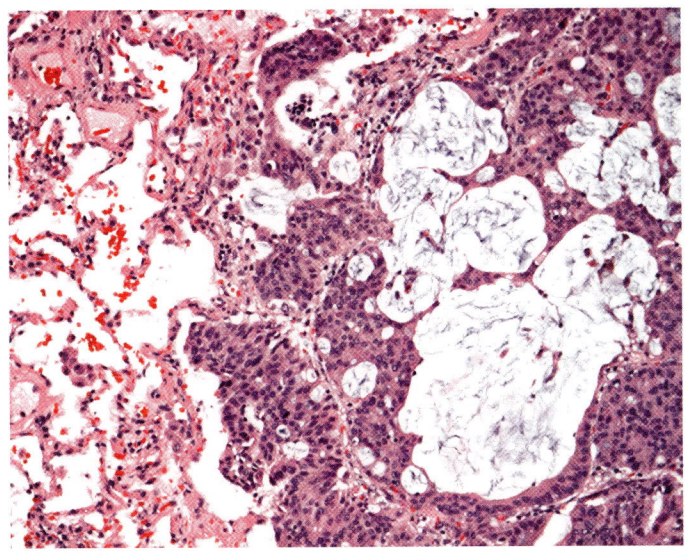

FIGURE 3.5. This medium-power view of a frozen section of a lung nodule shows an adenocarcinoma composed of relatively small, bland cells arranged in nests and small glands with small lakes of mucin. This cancer was excised to rule out primary lung carcinoma and was later confirmed to be metastatic carcinoma from a primary breast cancer that had been resected several years previously. When possible, having slides of a previous cancer biopsy or excision available for comparison at the time of frozen section can be very helpful in determining if a lung nodule has the histopathologic appearance of the previous cancer.

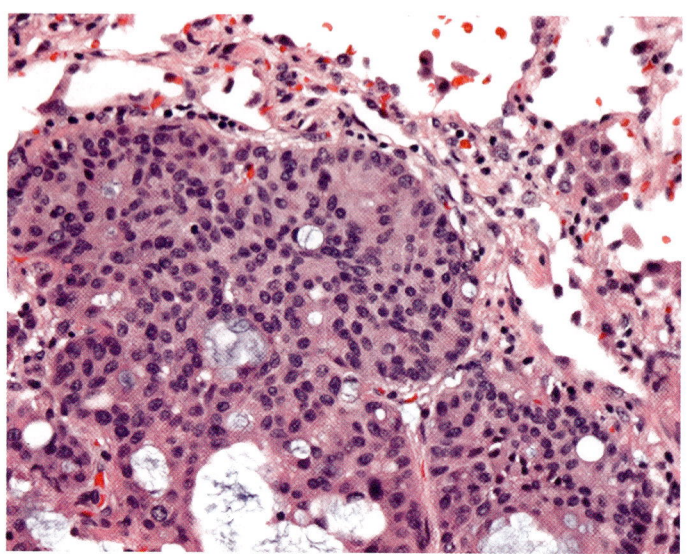

FIGURE 3.6. At high power the adenocarcinoma cells are relatively uniform and have comparatively round nuclei with only modest pleomorphism and only a moderately increased nucleus-to-cytoplasm ratio. When compared to nearby "normal" type II pneumocytes, endothelial cells, lymphocytes and macrophages, the cancer cells are only moderately larger. Although these features can be seen with other types of cancers, metastatic breast cancer is a consideration when an adenocarcinoma consists of nests or cords of relatively small, uniform, bland cells in contrast to a typical primary lung carcinoma which is likely to have considerable cytologic atypia and pleomorphism. In particular, metastatic lobular carcinoma may be deceptive on frozen section due to the modesty of the malignant features.

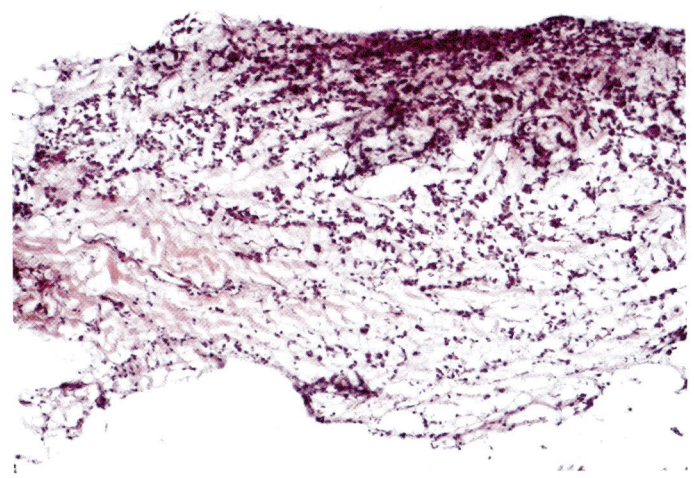

FIGURE 3.7. This frozen section of thickened pleura looks relatively innocuous at low power and demonstrates loose fibrous tissue with an infiltrate of relatively small, uniform, bland cells that suggest chronic inflammatory cells.

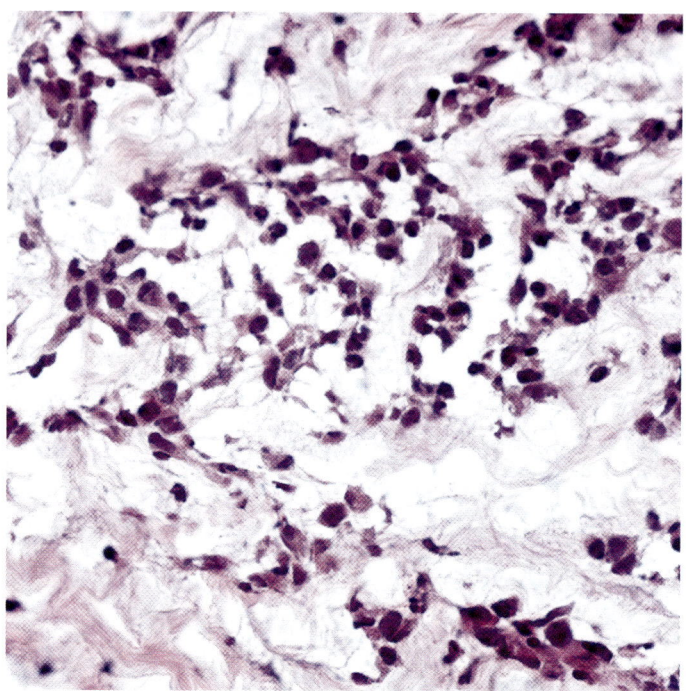

FIGURE 3.8. At higher power, the infiltrating cells are observed to be cohesive in cords and small clusters indicating that they are epithelial cells rather than lymphocytes. In addition, their nuclear chromatin is not that of lymphocytes. The infiltrating cells have comparatively uniform and round nuclei and have modest cytoplasm. This is an example of lobular carcinoma of the breast metastatic to the pleura which may mimic infiltrating lymphocytes at low power. Knowledge of the patient's history of lobular carcinoma is helpful in heightening suspicion for the correct diagnosis, but may not always be available. If the correct diagnosis remains ambiguous at frozen section, a final diagnosis can be deferred to permanent sections with confirmation by immunostains if indicated.

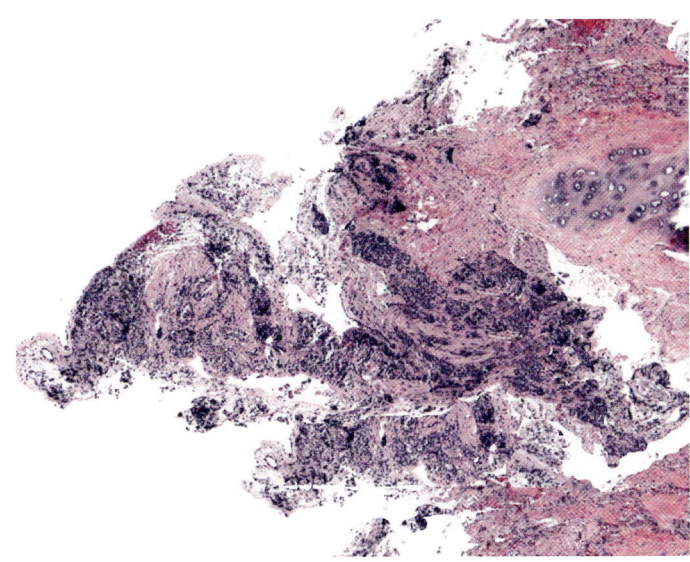

FIGURE 3.9. Low-power view of a frozen section of an endobronchial mass which was clinically suspicious for a primary bronchial neoplasm. Due in part to the blurring of detail by frozen section artifact, at low power the nests of cells are somewhat suggestive of a neuroendocrine carcinoma, possibly a carcinoid tumor because of the small gland pattern or a small cell carcinoma with pseudorosettes and crush artifact. This is a prostate carcinoma presenting as a solitary bronchial metastasis.

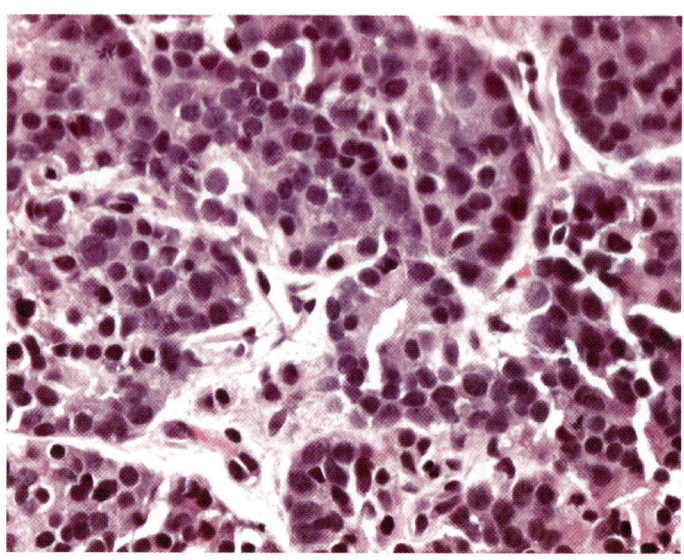

FIGURE 3.10. Higher-power view shows comparatively uniform, round nuclei and small glands of the metastatic prostate carcinoma in Fig. 3.9. Even at this power, a carcinoid tumor or other neuroendocrine neoplasm might be entertained when the only history is that of a solitary endobronchial mass. Nucleoli can be seen in some nuclei. Awareness that metastases can present as solitary masses, including as endobronchial masses is the first step in making the correct diagnosis at frozen section. The frozen section impression of metastatic prostate carcinoma can later be confirmed with immunostains of permanent sections if needed.

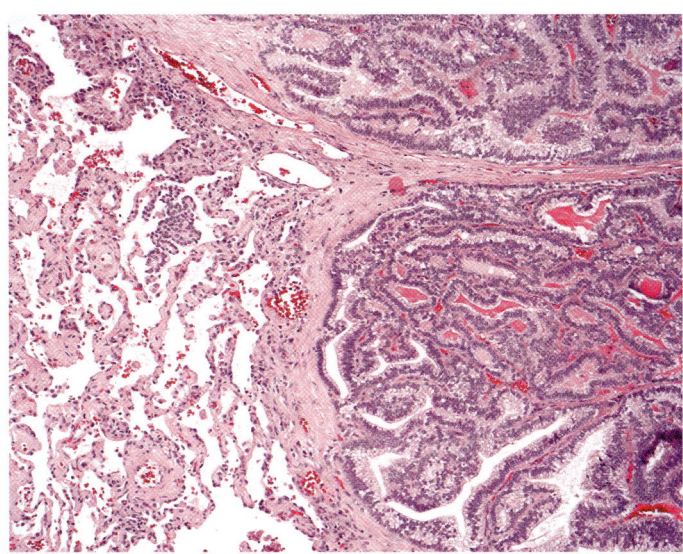

FIGURE 3.11. Frozen section of the interface between a focus of metastatic papillary adenocarcinoma of the thyroid and lung parenchyma. The differential diagnoses of papillary adenocarcinomas in the lung is given in Table 3.3 and, in addition to metastases from thyroid and other primaries, includes primary papillary adenocarcinoma of the lung and bronchioloalveolar carcinomas with papillary components. At the time of frozen section, the clinical impression and knowledge of previous primaries is important in arriving at the correct conclusion. It would be highly unusual for a papillary thyroid carcinoma to present as a metastasis to the lung with an occult primary.

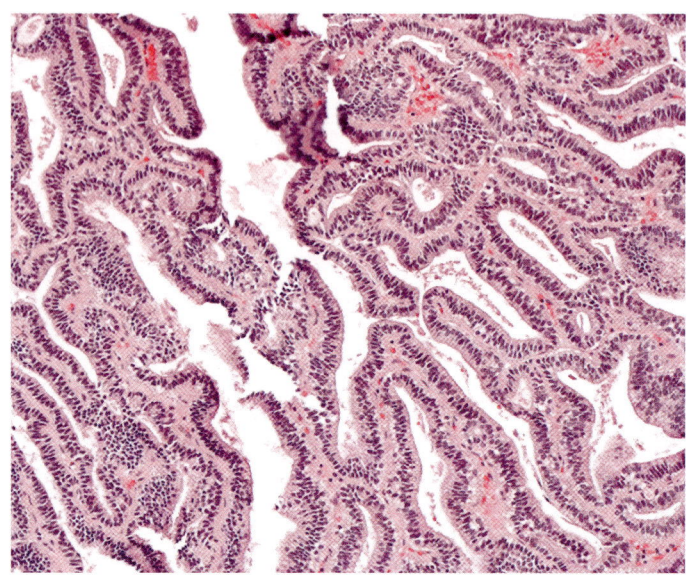

FIGURE 3.12. Higher-power view shows the relatively uniform columnar cells lining fibrovascular cores in a frozen section of a metastatic papillary thyroid adenocarcinoma.

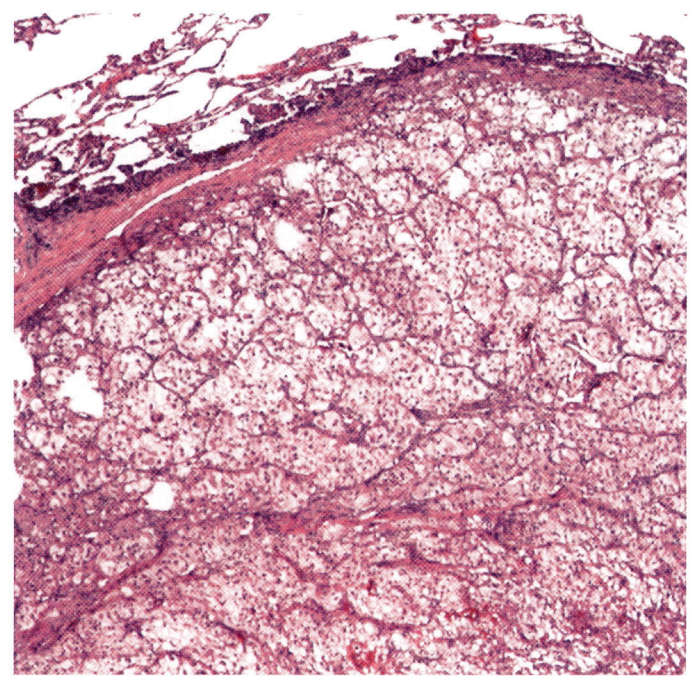

FIGURE 3.13. Frozen section at low power reveals a circumscribed nodule composed of clear cells consistent with metastatic renal cell carcinoma.

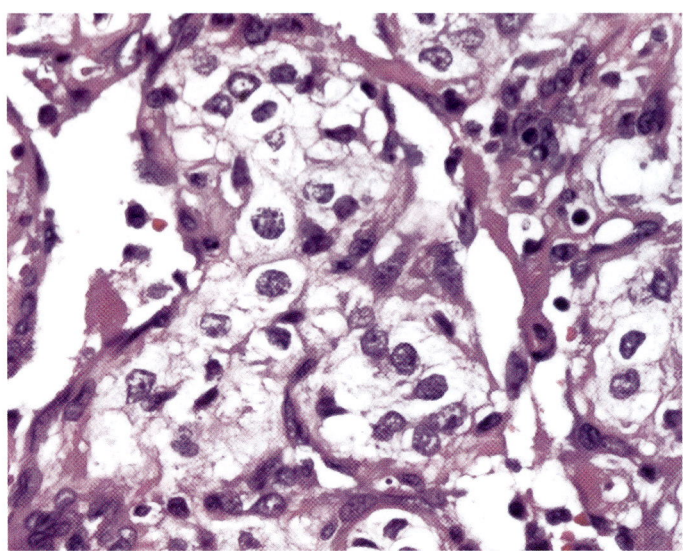

FIGURE 3.14. In contrast to primary clear cell carcinomas of the lung which tend to have pleomorphic nuclei, the nuclei of metastatic renal cell carcinoma cells, shown here at higher power, tend to be more uniform, round, and comparatively bland. In most cases, the history of a primary renal cell carcinoma is known at the time of frozen section of a solitary tumor metastasis in the lung.

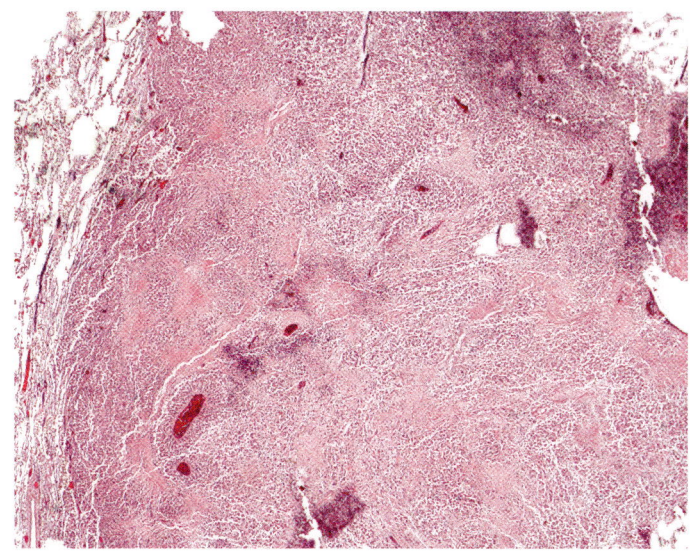

FIGURE 3.15. Low-power view of a frozen section of a lung mass consisting of sheets of discohesive malignant cells with abundant cytoplasm. The abundant eosinophilic cytoplasm gives the cells an epithelioid appearance. A carcinoma or epithelioid sarcoma might be suspected. This is a metastatic melanoma which is amelanotic. Metastatic melanomas are one of the great histopathologic mimickers of other cancers.

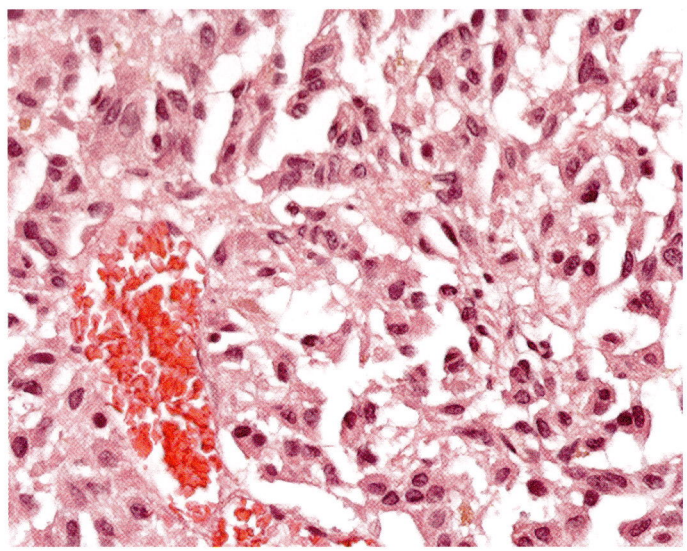

FIGURE 3.16. Higher-power view of Fig. 3.15 shows clusters of malignant "epithelioid" cells with abundant eosinophilic cytoplasm lacking melanin. The diagnosis of melanoma can be confirmed by immunostains performed later on the permanent sections, but the diagnosis of melanoma at frozen section requires appropriate suspicion if the clinical history of a previous melanoma primary is not available.

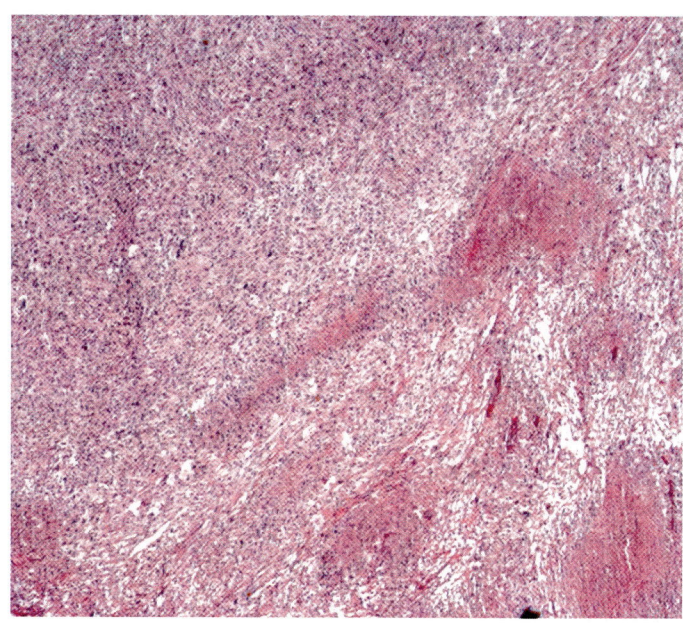

FIGURE 3.17. Low-power view of a sarcoma metastatic to the lung. At this power, the lesion is observed to be highly cellular with areas of hemorrhage. Most sarcomas in the lung are metastases and the previous primary site is often known. Primary sarcomas of the lung are rare, but do occur.

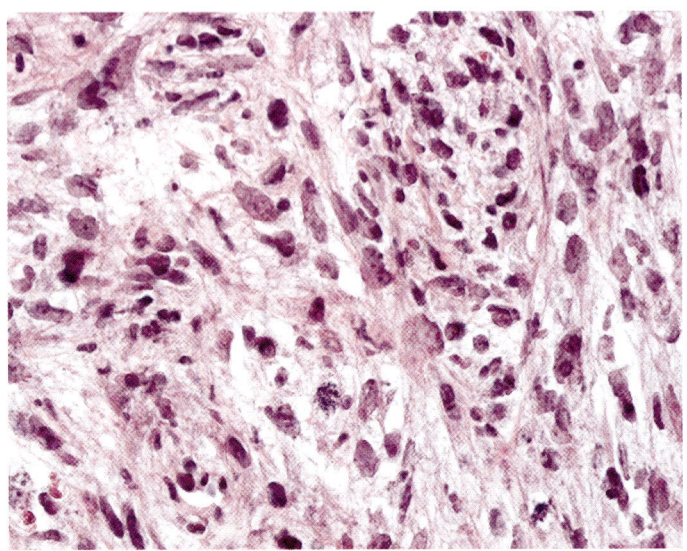

FIGURE 3.18. High-power view of Fig. 3.17 shows highly pleomorphic spindle cells, many with prominent nucleoli.

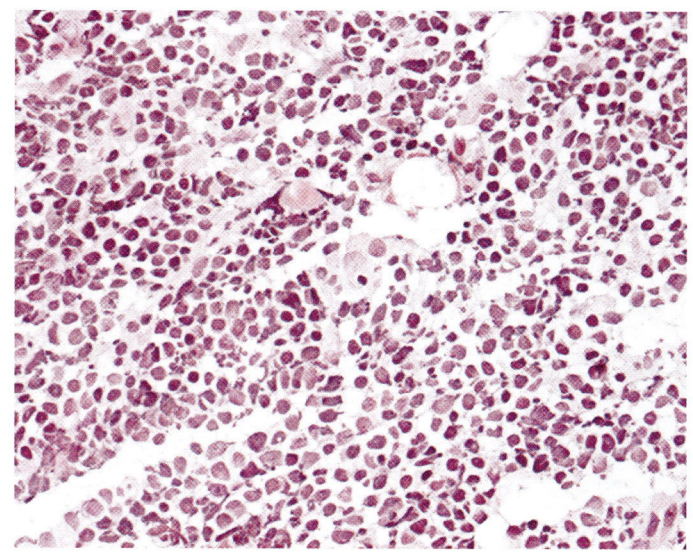

FIGURE 3.19. This frozen section of a mass in the lung consists of monotonous lymphoid cells. A diagnosis of "lymphoproliferative process–defer to permanent sections and special studies" was made on this frozen section and tissue was triaged for flow cytometry and other special studies. A diagnosis of lymphoma was later made based on the permanent sections and special studies. A definitive diagnosis of lymphoma may be difficult on frozen section and deferment of the final diagnosis is appropriate.

Chapter IV
Surgical Margins

BRONCHIAL SURGICAL MARGIN

Surgeons often request examination of the bronchial surgical margin for lobectomies and pneumonectomies performed for lung cancer to confirm that the surgeon has not cut across cancer in resecting the specimen. Relative to the common lung tumors, salivary gland-type tumors and carcinoid tumors have a higher incidence of positive margins. There are four patterns of microscopically positive bronchial margins to take into account: direct extension by overt cancer, lymphatic involvement with tumor, invasion of peribronchial tissues, and carcinoma in situ. It is important to note that residual carcinoma in situ at the bronchial margin has been shown to not alter patient survival, so while it should be noted by the pathologist if present, the decision to obtain additional bronchial margin is at the discretion of the surgeon.

The pathologist can cut a sliver of the bronchial surgical margin at the time of intraoperative consult and submit it en face for frozen section. Whether one prefers to place the "true" surgical margin face down or face up on the chuck is a personal preference. Generally, if one puts the true margin down and the first frozen section is positive for cancer, then one can cut additional sections for frozen section to observe whether the cancer disappears as one cuts deeper toward the true margin.

If cancer is observed involving the surgical margin, the surgeon must decide whether additional bronchus can be taken from a technical perspective. The surgical pathologist should be aware that bronchial margins may exhibit reactive atypia of the mucosa epithelium or the seromucinous bronchial glands which may occasionally suggest malignancy at frozen section. On occasion, frozen section of a bronchial surgical margin will show a tangential cut of the pseudostratified ciliated columnar epithelium which, when combined with frozen section artifact and/or reactive atypia, may initially suggest possible dysplasia or carcinoma-in-

T.C. Allen, P.T. Cagle, *Frozen Section Library: Lung*,
Frozen Section Library 1, DOI 10.1007/978-0-387-09573-8_4,
© Springer Science+Business Media, LLC 2009

situ (Figs. 4.1 through 4.3). Closer examination will disclose that the mucosa lacks nuclei with the degree of enlargement and cytologic pleomorphism found with dysplasia or carcinoma. In addition, the surface will typically display ciliated columnar epithelium that is unambiguously not dysplastic or neoplastic.

VASCULAR SURGICAL MARGIN

Ordinarily it is the bronchial margin that is sampled at frozen section for evaluation of the surgical margin in a lung cancer resection specimen. The vascular surgical margin can also be sampled if requested or grossly suspicious for abnormality.

OTHER SURGICAL MARGINS

With wedge resections, the pathologist can evaluate the parenchymal surgical margin which is typically stapled by the surgeon. Frozen section is performed to inform the surgeon whether or not the surgeon has cut across cancer in resecting the specimen.

Pleural margins may be sampled if the cancer is subpleural. Invasion through the visceral pleura should be reported to the surgeon. In cases of overt invasion through the pleura into adjacent chest wall or other structures, the surgeon is often already aware of the extent of disease. Whether or not additional surgery is performed when there is extension through the pleura depends on the objectives of the surgery and other clinical factors (Figs. 4.4 and 4.5).

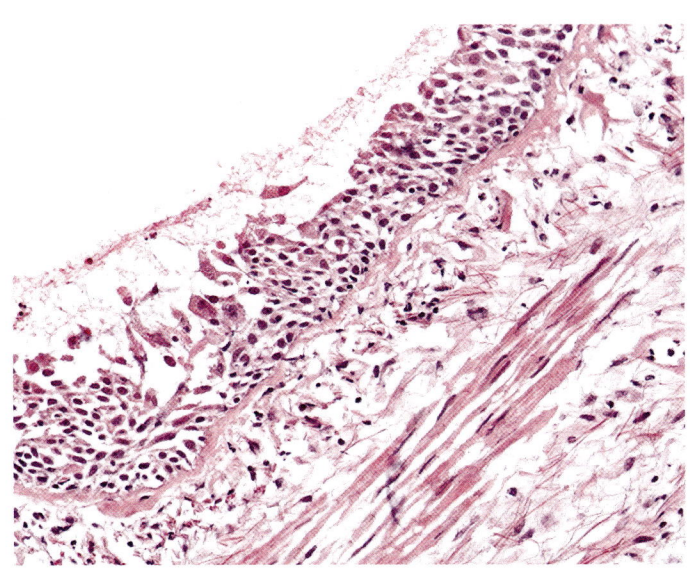

FIGURE 4.1. Tangential cut of bronchial margin frozen section gives an impression of increased cellularity and polygonal cells where columnar cells should be present. These features may suggest squamous metaplasia or even dysplasia depending on the presence of cytologic atypia. However, the cells display relatively small, cytologically bland nuclei and ciliated columnar cells on the surface indicating that the features suggesting abnormality are the result of a tangential cut of the pseudostratified ciliated columnar epithelium.

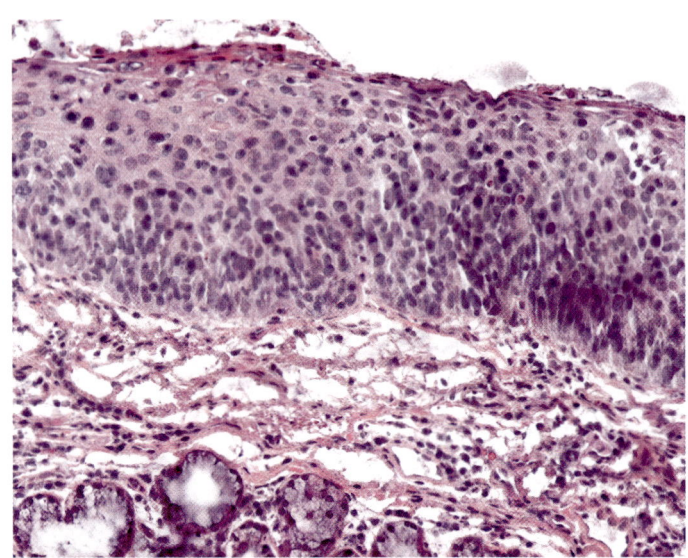

FIGURE 4.2. In this frozen section, the bronchial margin mucosa shows full-thickness severely dysplastic squamous epithelium or carcinoma-in-situ. No invasive malignancy is identified. Although the surgeon should be made aware of this finding and may elect to take additional bronchial margin, leaving carcinoma-in-situ behind at the bronchial margin does not alter patient survival.

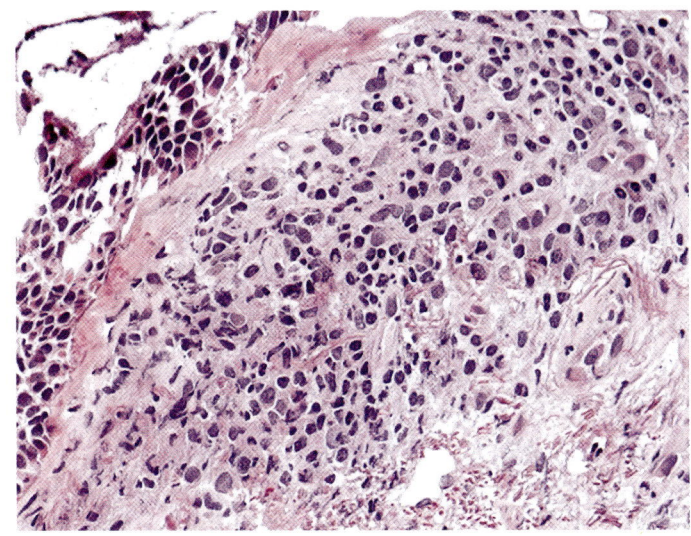

FIGURE 4.3. This frozen section of a bronchial margin is positive for invasive non-small cell carcinoma which is extending in the submucosal bronchial tissue. If technical factors permit, the surgeon will take additional bronchial margin to avoid leaving invasive cancer behind at the surgical margin.

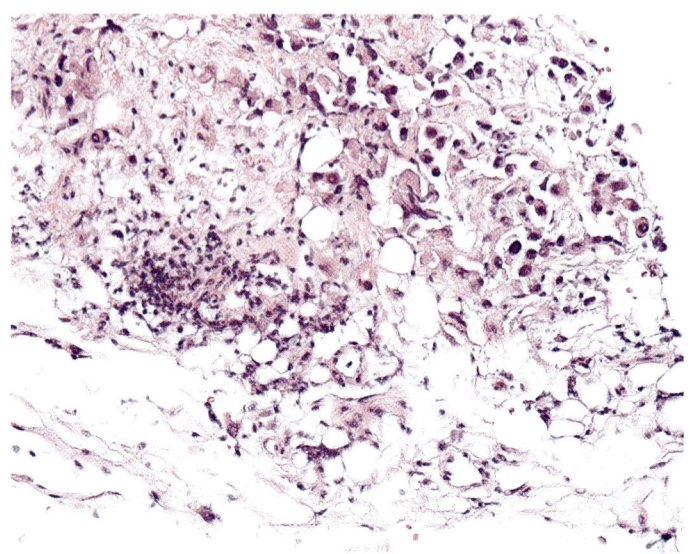

FIGURE 4.4. High-power view of a frozen section of a pleural margin shows nests of non-small cell carcinoma cells extending from a fibrous adhesion of the visceral pleura and invading into parietal pleural fat. In this situation, the surgeon likely suspects extension of the tumor through the visceral pleura and into the parietal pleura and this suspicion is confirmed at frozen section. Depending on various surgical and clinical factors, it may be necessary to leave residual tumor at the positive pleural margin behind in this situation.

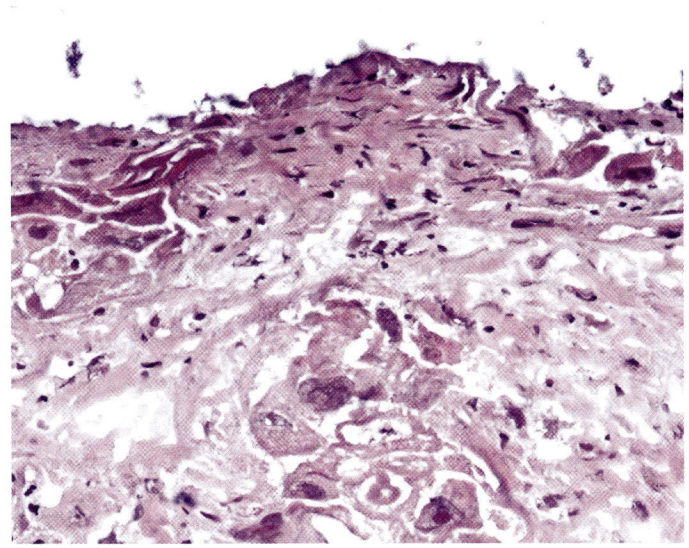

FIGURE 4.5. High-power view of a positive pleural margin on frozen section shows tiny groups and individual non-small cell carcinoma cells extending near and into the visceral pleural surface from an underlying carcinoma in the lung parenchyma.

Chapter V
Benign Focal Lesions

Benign focal lesions are occasionally sampled and sent for frozen section primarily to rule out malignancy. Granulomas and focal organizing pneumonias make up most of these lesions, less frequently hamartomas, scars, and other benign masses. Most of these are incidental findings on imaging studies and typically the surgeon suspects the true diagnosis, but wants reassurance that additional surgery is not needed before wakening the patient. In some cases, an incidental mass has been observed for a period of time by imaging techniques and has enlarged, suggesting that it may be a neoplasm.

Gross examination of most benign focal lesions will suggest the correct diagnosis. Infectious granulomas often have firm, sometimes calcified rims with caseous necrosis. Hamartomas usually have a cartilaginous cut surface and abscesses contain purulent material. These gross features often contrast to the firm tan-white tissue of a carcinoma. However, carcinomas may also exhibit central necrosis, adjacent pneumonia, or other gross features that may overlap with the gross features of various benign focal lesions. Therefore, although very helpful in the majority of cases, gross features may sometimes be equivocal.

It may be preferable to perform a touch or scrape preparation of a caseating nodule that grossly appears to be an infectious granuloma. This allows an intraoperative diagnosis with minimal exposure of personnel to the potential infectious agent and without contaminating a cryostat that will then require decontamination.

Examples of the more common benign focal lesions potentially encountered at frozen section are illustrated in Figs. 5.1 through 5.20.

T.C. Allen, P.T. Cagle, *Frozen Section Library: Lung*,
Frozen Section Library 1, DOI 10.1007/978-0-387-09573-8_5,
© Springer Science+Business Media, LLC 2009

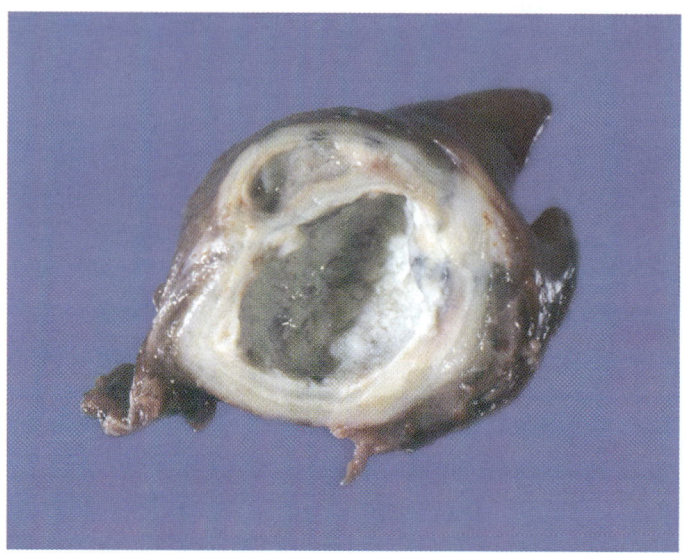

FIGURE 5.1. Gross appearance of an excised pulmonary granuloma shows a central cavity containing residual pasty-white necrotic material (caseous necrosis). The wall of the granuloma consists of dense yellow-tan-to-ivory fibrous tissue. The gross appearance of the granuloma has some similarities to the cavitary squamous cell carcinoma in Fig. 5.2, although there are some differences. Suspicion of an infectious granuloma based on the gross appearance of the specimen raises concerns about contaminating personnel and cryostats with infectious organisms if the suspicion proves correct. Therefore, touch preparations or scrape preparations may be preferred over frozen section to reach a diagnosis.

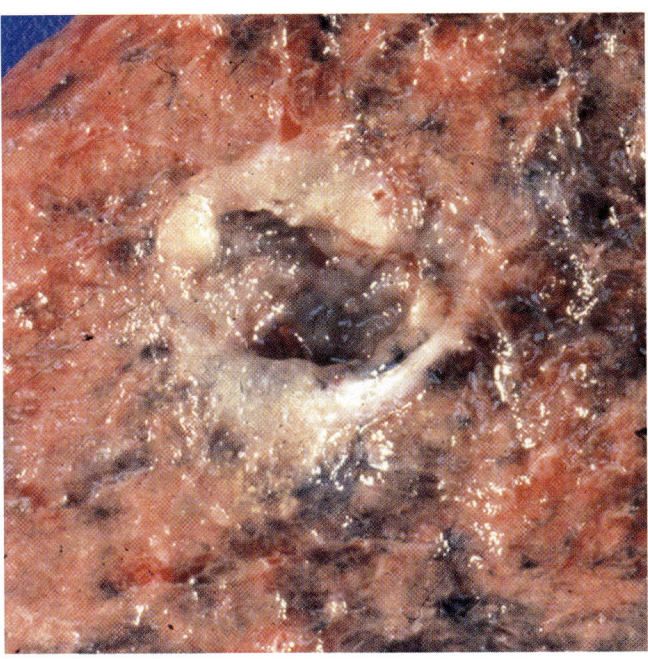

FIGURE 5.2. For comparison, gross appearance of a resected cavitary squamous cell carcinoma resembles the cavitary granuloma in Fig. 5.1. The wall of the cavity within the squamous cell carcinoma has a fleshier, less fibrous consistency in this case. Frozen section or a touch or scrape preparation may be required to confirm whether a cavitary lesion is a granuloma or cancer.

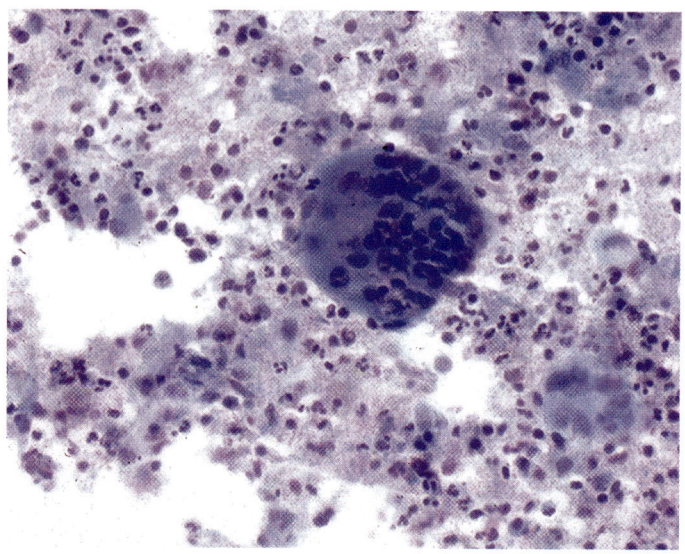

FIGURE 5.3. Scrape preparation from the cut surface of a granuloma shows histiocytes, neutrophils, and a multinucleated giant cell. The histiocytes have round smooth-bordered nuclei and a low nucleus-to-cytoplasm ratio consistent with benign cells. The multinucleated giant cell also has round, smooth-bordered, small nuclei indicating that it is a benign cell rather than a multinucleated malignant cell. The size of the neutrophils provides a convenient comparison for the size of the nuclei of the histiocytes and giant cell.

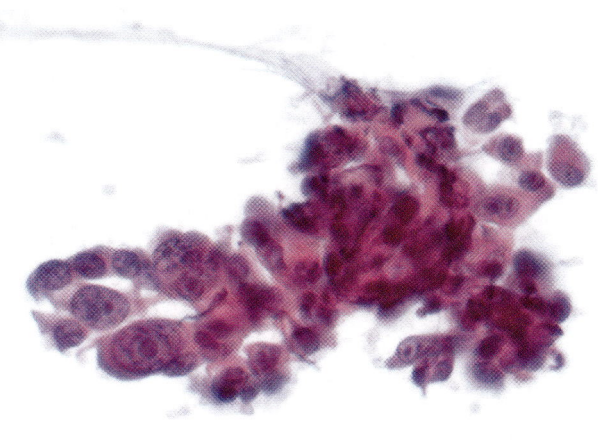

FIGURE 5.4. Scrape preparation from the cut surface of a non-small cell carcinoma shows cohesive epithelial cells with high nucleus-to-cytoplasm ratio and enlarged nucleoli consistent with malignant cells. These carcinoma cells are a sharp contrast to the "normal" inflammatory cells and benign multinucleated giant cell seen in the scrape preparation from the granuloma.

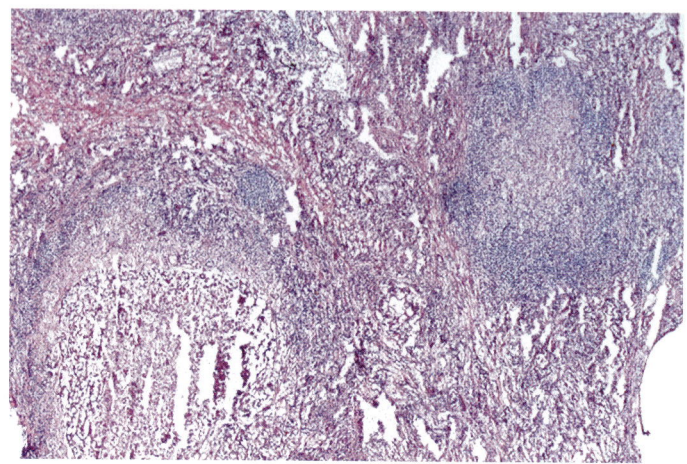

FIGURE 5.5. Low-power view of lung tissue with granulomas. Aggregates of inflammatory cells and fibrosis are recognizable, and the granuloma in the lower left has central necrosis. In addition to the frozen section artifact that blurs some of the details, there are tissue tears in the areas of necrosis. Necrosis does not cut well at frozen section and tissue tears like this are often seen in the necrosis. Recut of the section can be attempted if the amount of tearing is significant enough to obscure details. Well-formed granulomas with central necrosis are likely to represent infection, including fungus and mycobacteria.

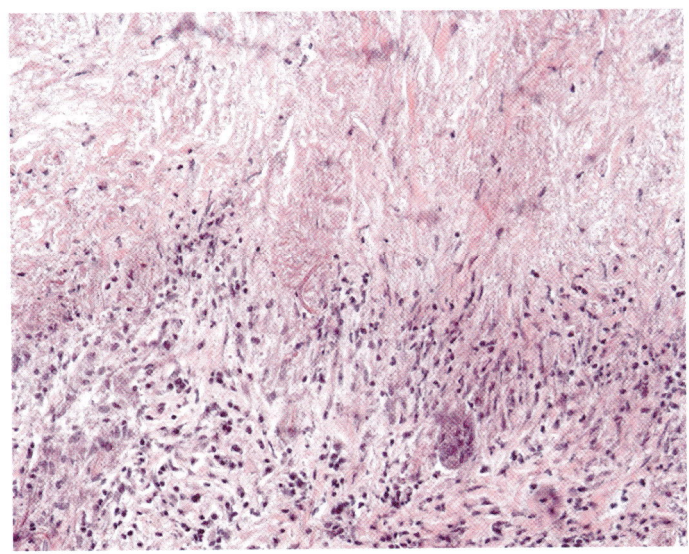

Figure 5.6. Higher-power view shows edge of a necrotizing granuloma including caseous necrosis and a rim of palisading epithelioid histiocytes and a multinucleated giant cell. Occasionally larger fungal organisms such as *Aspergillus* hyphae can be seen on H&E-stained frozen sections or touch or scrape preparations. Often organisms are not seen and necrotizing granulomas should be assumed to represent infection and proper precautions taken even when organisms are not apparent. If tissue samples have not already been taken for fungal, mycobacterial, and other appropriate cultures by the surgeon, the pathologist should submit tissue for this purpose.

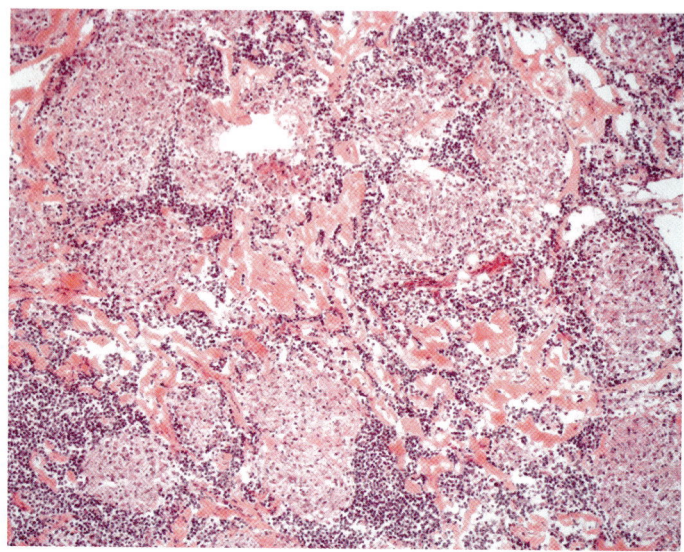

FIGURE 5.7. Low-power view of a frozen section of lung tissue shows multiple, well-formed granulomas without necrosis. Sarcoidosis is in the differential diagnosis for this type of granuloma, but infection cannot be ruled out by the histopathologic appearance alone. Proper precautions and microbiologic cultures should be taken in case fungal or mycobacterial infection is present.

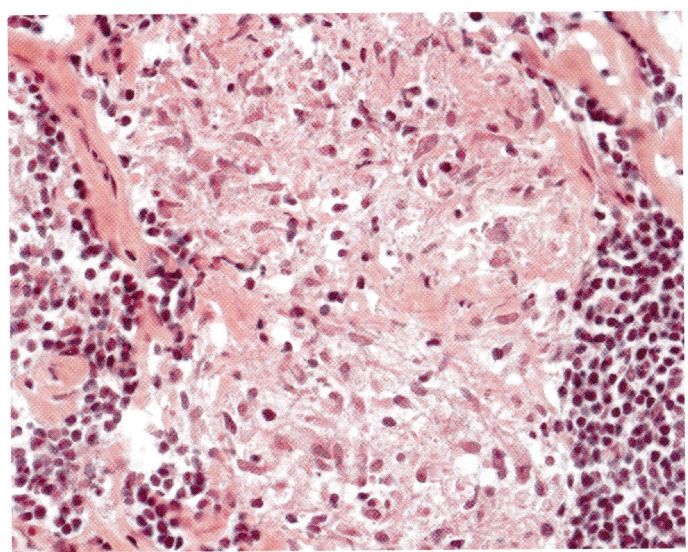

FIGURE 5.8. At higher power, the epithelioid histiocytes composing the granulomas are observed to have features of benign cells including low nucleus-to-cytoplasm ratio and round, regular nuclei. As a result of normal variation combined with frozen section artifact, individual nuclei may appear slightly enlarged and irregular and nucleoli may be observed in individual histiocyte nuclei at high power. However, the degree of atypia of individual cells and the collective appearance of the cells is not that of carcinoma cells.

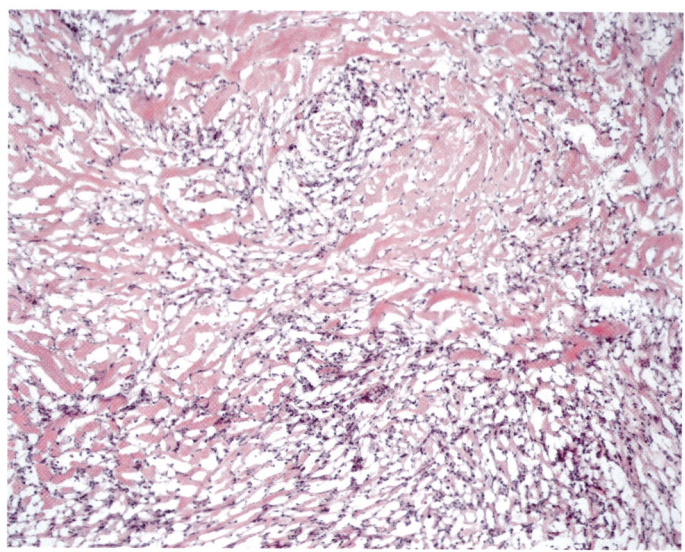

FIGURE 5.9. Pulmonary hyalinizing granuloma is rare and presents as a lung nodule. Especially when in association with sclerosing mediastinitis, it may clinically resemble a lung cancer with mediastinal extension or metastasis. This medium-power frozen section shows the characteristic thick "ropey" collagen and infiltrate of lymphocytes. No malignant cells are seen despite the possible clinical impression.

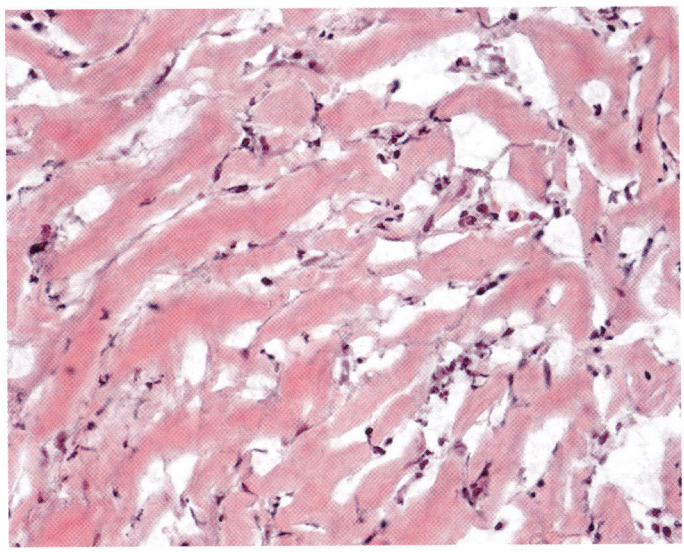

FIGURE 5.10. Higher-power view of the dense, acellular, "ropey" collagen bundles of a pulmonary hyalinizing granuloma. Sclerosing mediastinitis has the same histopathologic appearance and may occur in the same patient suggesting an infiltrative neoplasm clinically. No malignant cells are present and the intraoperative report from the pathologist can spare the patient further surgery. Many of these cases are found to be associated with *Histoplasma*.

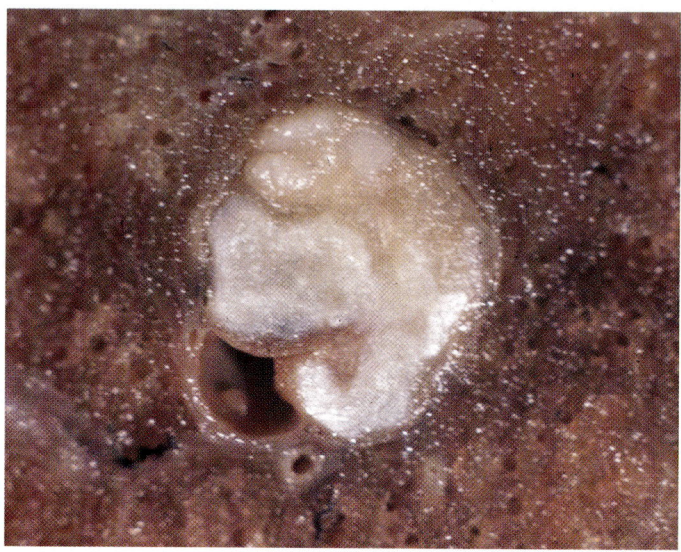

FIGURE 5.11. Gross appearance of a pulmonary hamartoma shows a well-circumscribed mass with cartilaginous consistency. The hamartoma or mesenchymoma is considered the most frequent benign neoplasm of the lung. The diagnosis is usually apparent from imaging studies. Most have a significant cartilaginous component which is evident on gross examination, but the lesions may have other soft tissue elements which may occasionally be predominant. A minority of hamartomas are endobronchial masses rather than peripheral nodules.

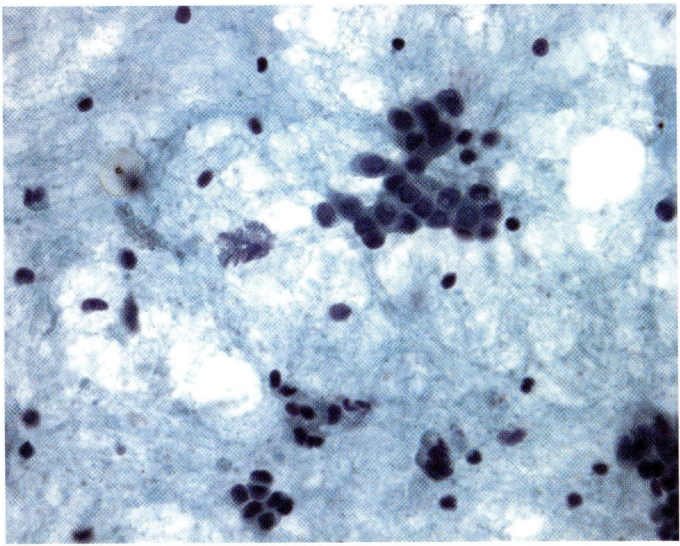

FIGURE 5.12. Scrape preparation from an intraoperative consultation shows clusters of benign epithelial cells representing entrapped pulmonary epithelium from a hamartoma.

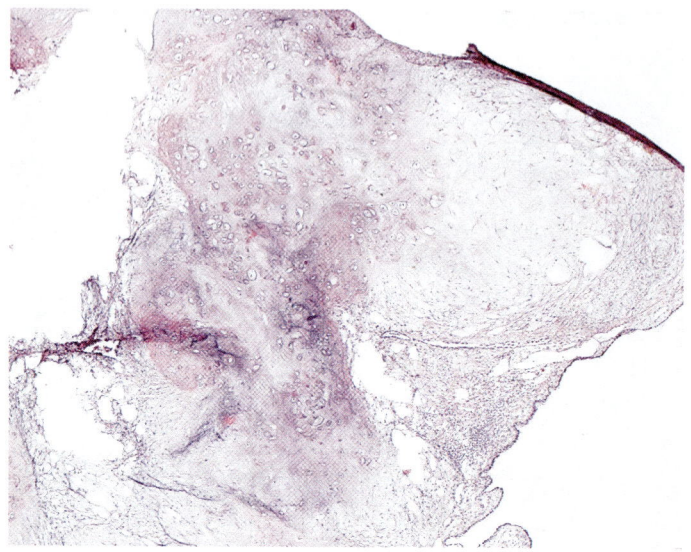

FIGURE 5.13. Low–power view of a frozen section shows a hamartoma composed of a cartilaginous mass with a cleft lined by benign epithelial cells.

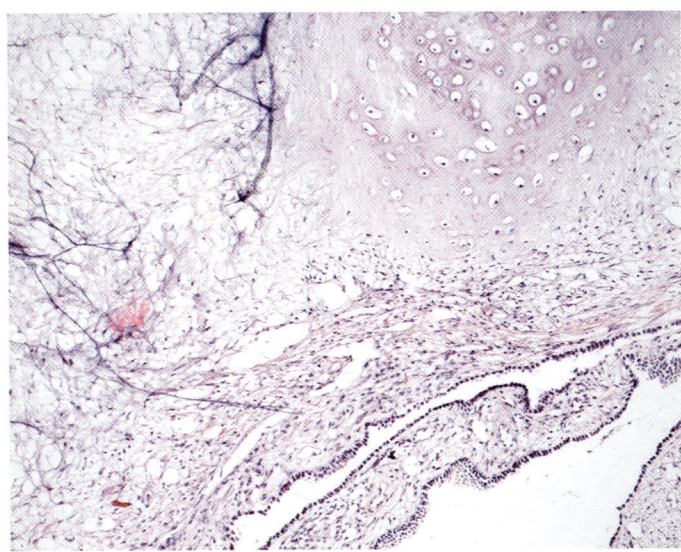

FIGURE 5.14. High-power view of a frozen section of a hamartoma shows a cleft lined by a single row of uniform cuboidal cells with small round nuclei. These features are benign and the epithelial cells are considered entrapped epithelium and not a neoplastic component.

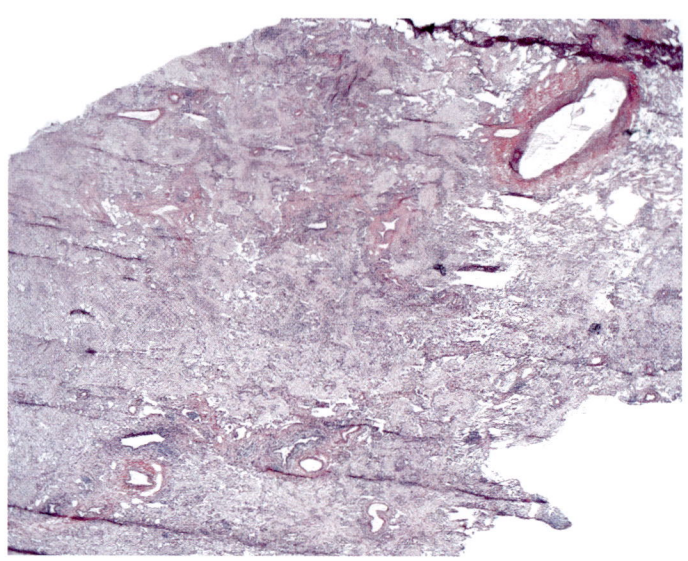

FIGURE 5.15. Low–power view of a frozen section of a lung mass shows interstitial infiltrates of blue inflammatory cells and filling of alveolar spaces and ducts with pale eosinophilic granulation tissue. This consolidated appearance of the lung parenchyma at low power is consistent with an organizing pneumonia.

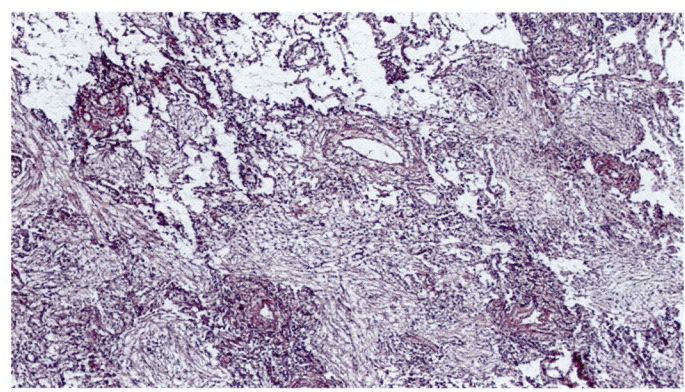

FIGURE 5.16. At higher power, despite blurring of details by frozen section artifact, structures such as blood vessels and alveolar septa can be discerned. The alveolar spaces are filled by a loose, myxoid stroma containing wavy fibroblasts. Smatterings of small round blue cells representing lymphocytes are focally present around blood vessels and elsewhere in the interstitium. No nests or clusters of cytologically malignant cells are seen at this medium power.

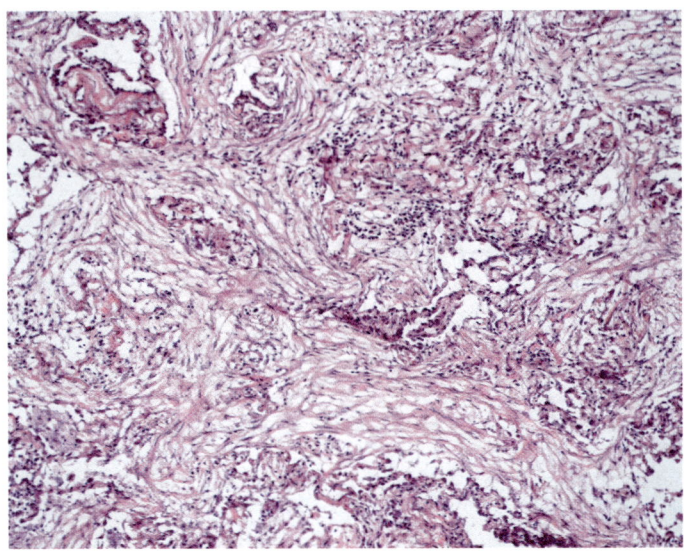

FIGURE 5.17. High–power view shows that the granulation tissue filling the alveolar spaces consists of wavy collagen and fibroblasts with small benign nuclei against a vacuolated background. Also present is denser, darker collagen of pre-existing interstitium and small, round, blue lymphocytes. These are features of organizing pneumonia at frozen section of a lung mass excised to rule out malignancy.

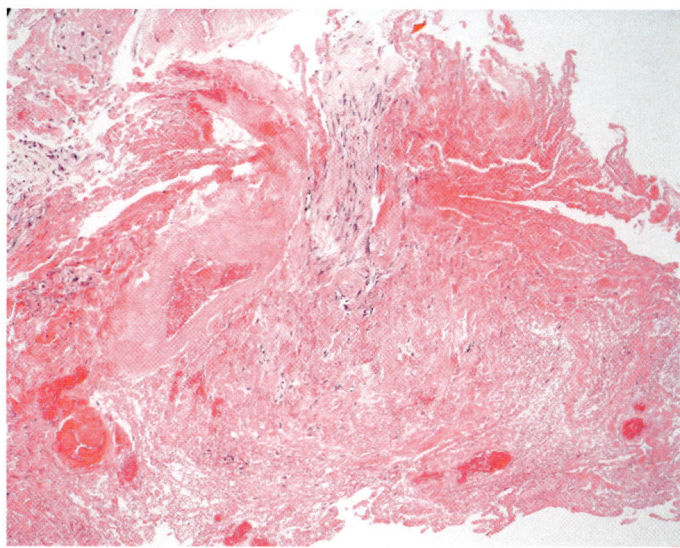

FIGURE 5.18. Low–power view of frozen section of a pulmonary infarct shows eosinophilic necrotic parenchyma and dark red of congested vessels and hemorrhage. This infarct appeared radiologically as a mass and frozen section was performed to rule out malignant neoplasm.

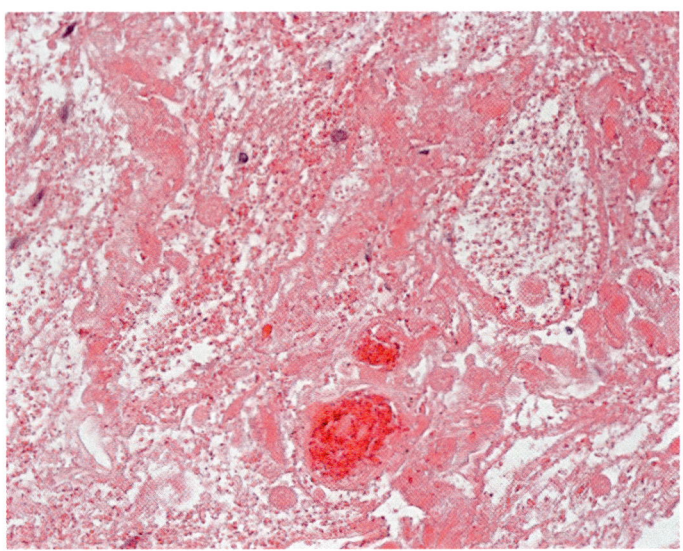

FIGURE 5.19. At higher power, the eosinophilic ghosts or outlines of pulmonary structures such as alveolar septa and blood vessels can be recognized accompanied by congested vessels and fresh hemorrhage. These findings are consistent with a pulmonary infarct. No malignant cells are identified.

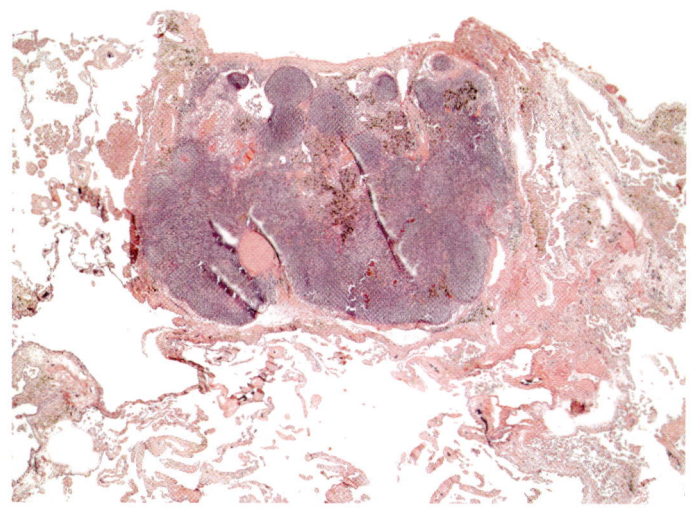

FIGURE 5.20. Low-power view of a frozen section of an intraparenchymal lymph node which presented as a lung mass and was excised to rule out cancer. Histologic features of a lymph node are readily observed including lymphoid tissue, capsule, and sinus histiocytes containing pigment.

Chapter VI
Wedge Biopsy for Diffuse Lung Diseases

Wedge biopsy via thoracoscopic biopsy or open lung biopsy is occasionally performed to obtain tissue for the diagnosis of a diffuse lung disease. A wedge biopsy is more invasive and has higher risks of morbidity and mortality than other diagnostic procedures and the so only a minority of patients have circumstances that cause their pulmonologist or other clinician to request a wedge biopsy. In general, the patient is either severely acutely ill or is ill with a chronic disease that has eluded definitive diagnosis by more conservative means (clinical tests, imaging, cytology, transbronchial biopsy) and not responded to empirical treatments.

Since the decision to obtain a wedge biopsy has significant potential consequences and the patient is already in a difficult clinical situation, frozen section may be performed to confirm that the lung tissue sampled is appropriate for diagnostic purposes. Specifically, the intent of the frozen section is not to provide a diagnosis of a diffuse disease at the time of frozen section, but rather confirm that diagnostic tissue has been obtained that can be analyzed on permanent sections. Presumably if the wedge biopsy has not sampled appropriate or adequate tissue for diagnosis, then additional tissue should be sampled.

To address the question of whether the wedge biopsy represents diagnostic tissue, it is important for the pathologist to obtain clinical information from the pulmonologist or other informed clinician. The sample's appropriateness depends on the clinical differential diagnosis and questions to be answered. In some cases, tissue for microbiologic cultures or other special studies may also be obtained at the time of wedge biopsy.

A description of the histopathologic features of all diffuse lung diseases is beyond the scope of this book. There are some basic concepts that the pathologist performing the frozen section will find helpful. Since the patient may be very ill, the surgeon may be hurried into taking a sample that is not representative of the disease

T.C. Allen, P.T. Cagle, *Frozen Section Library: Lung*,
Frozen Section Library 1, DOI 10.1007/978-0-387-09573-8_6,
© Springer Science+Business Media, LLC 2009

process; for example, the lingula often protrudes as an easy target for excision, but may not be representative of the active disease. As much as possible, the surgeon should be encouraged to sample areas of active disease and rather than any lung tissue that happens to be surgically convenient. Obviously, normal lung tissue or tissue with end-stage fibrosis is not diagnostic. Tissue with active inflammation, acute injury, organization, or other features within the clinical differential diagnosis is necessary. Usually all that is required at frozen section is for the pathologist to confirm that lung tissue with active diffuse disease is present and further diagnosis is deferred for permanent sections.

In reviewing the frozen section for features of disease, the pathologist should be careful to avoid misinterpreting reactive atypia for malignancy as discussed in Chapter I. Rarely, diffuse interstitial lung disease is the result of lymphangitic spread of a cancer which may be sampled on frozen section. Examples of wedge biopsies that may be submitted for frozen section are illustrated in Figs. 6.1 through 6.5.

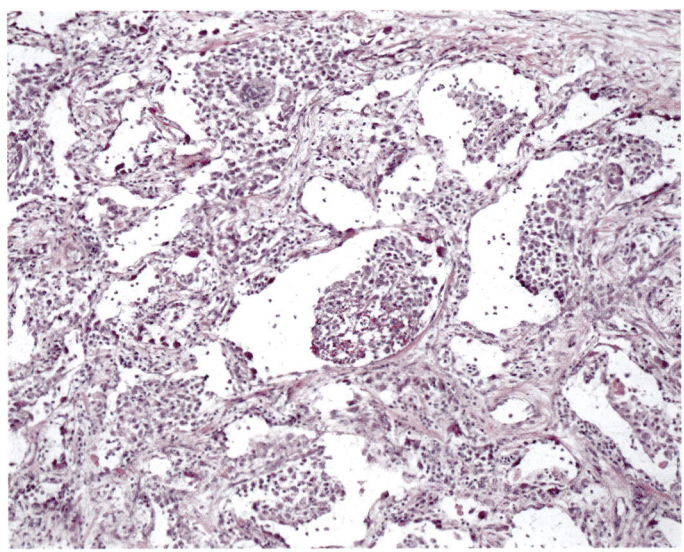

FIGURE 6.1. Medium-power view of a frozen section for a diffuse lung disease shows intra-alveolar collections of macrophages and eosinophils and interstitial thickening by edema, granulation tissue, and lymphocytes. This is clearly active disease and suitable specimen for evaluation on permanent sections later. This was later diagnosed as eosinophilic pneumonia.

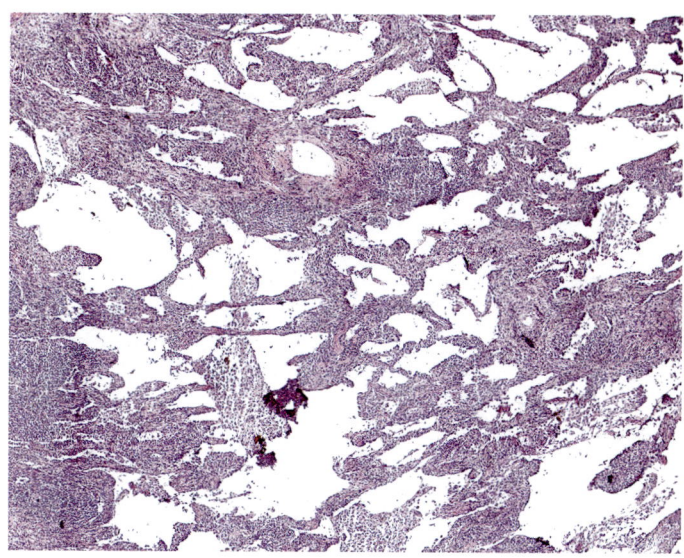

FIGURE 6.2. Low-power view of a frozen section shows a wedge biopsy of lung parenchyma in which there are diffuse interstitial lymphocytic infiltrates. The wedge biopsy consists of lung tissue with active disease appropriate for further evaluation on permanent sections.

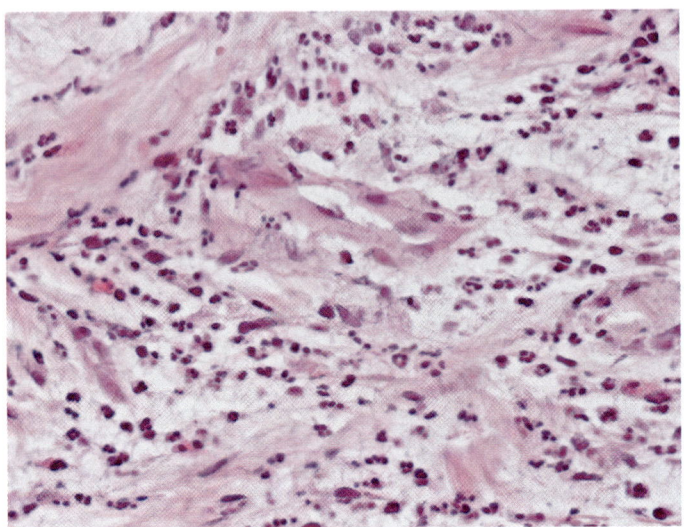

FIGURE 6.3. High-power view from a wedge biopsy frozen section containing neutrophils and granulation tissue. These features are consistent with an infection and, in addition, confirm that tissue with active disease has been sampled. Tissue should also be sent for microbiologic cultures.

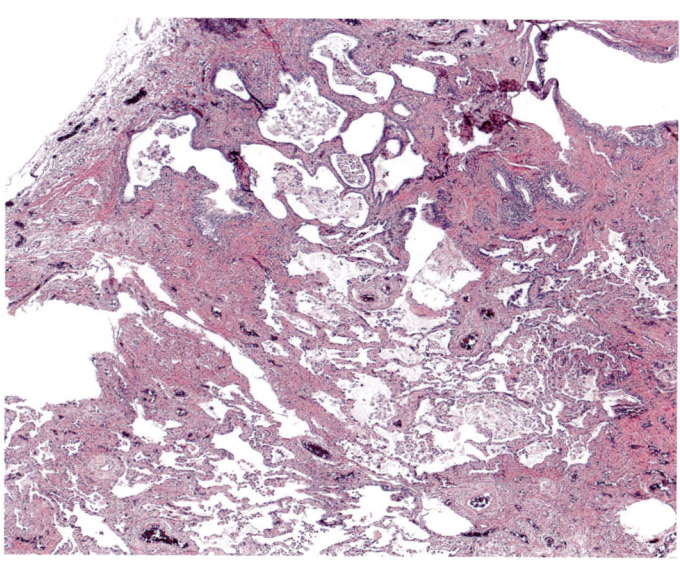

FIGURE 6.4. There is considerable mature fibrosis in this wedge biopsy reviewed at frozen section. Biopsies of end-stage fibrosis are not of diagnostic utility because they do not represent diagnosable areas of active disease. However, it is important for the pathologist to know the clinical differential diagnosis and questions to be answered before making a decision on the suitability of the biopsy on frozen section. This biopsy was performed for a chronic idiopathic interstitial fibrosis that had a slightly atypical pattern on imaging studies. This biopsy shows a patchy pattern of fibrosis suggestive of usual interstitial pneumonia on frozen section and the pathologist indicated to the surgeon that appropriate tissue had been sampled. Other features of usual interstitial pneumonia such as fibroblast foci were identified on the permanent sections.

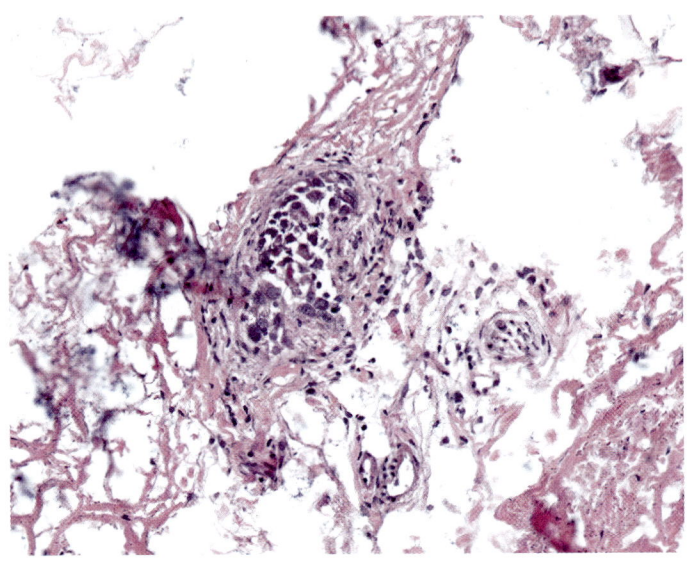

FIGURE 6.5. This patient presented with an interstitial infiltrate and underwent wedge biopsy when less invasive studies failed to confirm a specific disease. At frozen section, the patient was found to have lymphangitic spread of carcinoma. In this figure, there is a vessel filled with cytologically malignant carcinoma cells.

Chapter VII
Lymph Nodes

The pathologist is often asked to assess by frozen section whether mediastinal or other biopsied lymph nodes are negative for metastatic lung carcinoma before the surgeon proceeds with a lung cancer resection. If the biopsied lymph nodes are found to be positive for metastatic carcinoma, the surgeon typically does not proceed with the resection. Usually the status of the sampled lymph nodes is

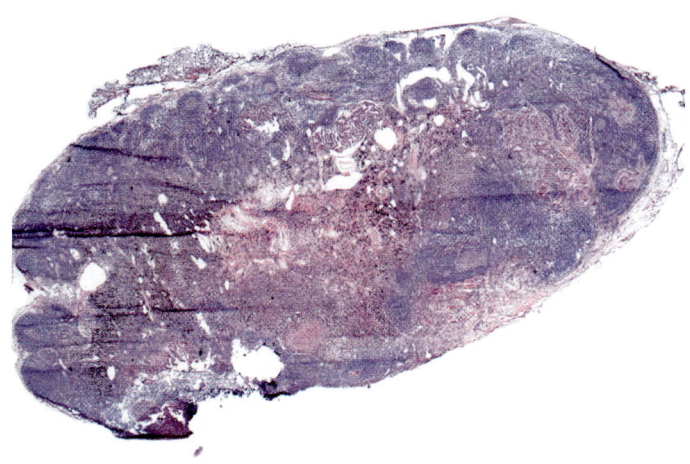

FIGURE 7.1. Low–power view of a mediastinal lymph node at frozen section. The lymph node consists of many blue-staining lymphocytes with a surrounding capsule and paler, more eosinophilic central area of histiocytes. There are distinct pink-purple foci of metastatic carcinoma in the right-hand third of the lymph node and a subcapsular focus along the right lower edge. Most lymph node metastases are apparent at low power.

T.C. Allen, P.T. Cagle, *Frozen Section Library: Lung*,
Frozen Section Library 1, DOI 10.1007/978-0-387-09573-8_7,
© Springer Science+Business Media, LLC 2009

unambiguous on the frozen section, but lymph nodes from cancer patients may contain granulomas or other pathology that should be distinguished from metastatic carcinoma. The pathologist should keep in mind that granulomas may also clinically mimic metastases, for example, resulting in a positive PET scan, which may further bias interpretation of an abnormal lymph node in a cancer patient. Frozen sections of lymph nodes with metastatic lung carcinoma are illustrated in Figs. 7.1 through 7.4.

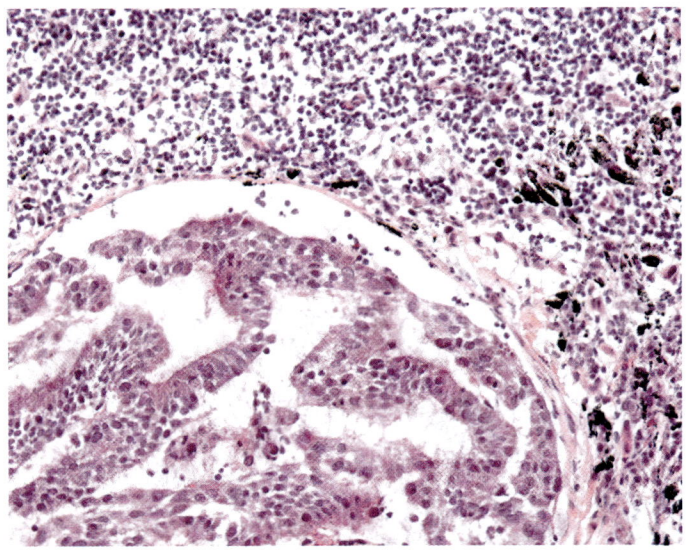

FIGURE 7.2. High-power view shows metastatic adenocarcinoma in a mediastinal lymph node sampled at frozen section. The contrast between the focus of metastatic adenocarcinoma and the lymphocytes and other normal structures is conspicuous. The black pigment is anthracotic pigment which has traveled via lymphatics from alveoli into which it was inhaled. Anthracotic pigment is commonly seen in hilar and mediastinal lymph nodes in city dwellers, smokers, and others with exposure to carbon particles in inhaled air and typically seen in frozen sections of these lymph nodes.

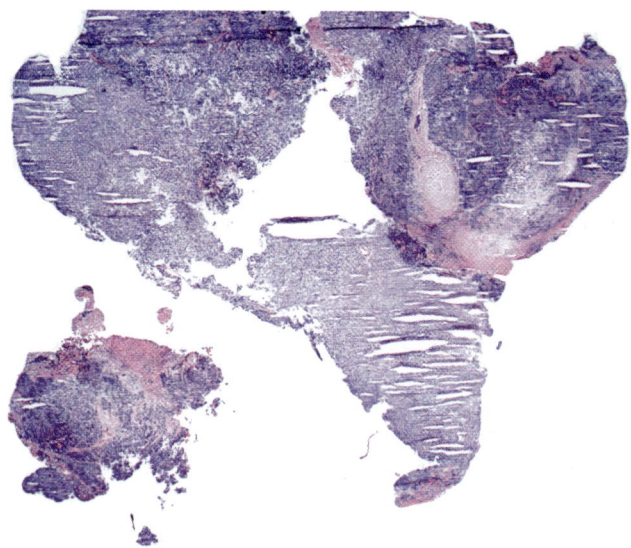

FIGURE 7.3. Small cell carcinoma often metastasizes to hilar and mediastinal lymph nodes. In the low-power view of the frozen section of this mediastinal lymph node, the cells in the node are small, round, blue cells, superficially resembling lymphocytes. However, effacement of the normal nodal architecture, crush artifact, and focal necrosis suggest that the lymph node has been replaced by tissue other than normal lymphocytes.

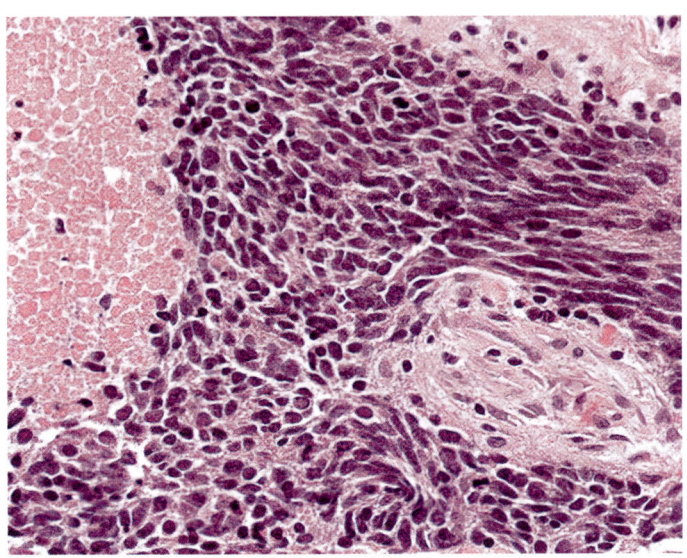

FIGURE 7.4. Higher-power view of Fig. 7.3 demonstrates polygonal-to-spindle cells with scant cytoplasm, stippled, salt and pepper chromatin, nuclear molding, and necrosis. The cells are 2–3 times the size of lymphocytes. The cells are those of metastatic small cell carcinoma and are not lymphocytes.

Suggested Reading

Cagle PT. Carcinoma of the lung. In: *Pathology of the Lung*, 3rd ed, Churg AM, Myers JL, Tazelaar HD, Wright JL, editors, pp. 413–479. Thieme Medical Publishers: New York, 2005.

Fraire AE. Non-malignant versus malignant proliferations on lung biopsy. In: *Diagnostic Pulmonary Pathology*, Cagle PT, editor, pp. 525–545. Marcel Dekker: New York, 2000.

Laga AC, Allen T, Ostrowski M, Cagle PT. Reactive changes, nonspecific findings and age-related changes. In: *The Color Atlas and Text of Pulmonary Pathology*, Cagle PT (editor-in-chief), pp. 25–27. Lippincott Williams and Wilkins: New York, 2005.

Marchevsky AM, Changsri C, Gupta I, Fukker C, Houch W, McKenna RJ, Jr. Frozen section diagnoses of small pulmonary nodules: accuracy and clinical implications. Ann Thotac Surg. 2004;78:1755–1760.

Nashef SA, Kakadellis JG, Hasleton PS, Whittaker JS, Gregory CM, Jones MT. Histological examination of preoperative frozen sections in suspected lung cancer. Thorax. 1993;48(4):388–389.

Sienko A, Allen TC, Zander DS, Cagle PT. Frozen section of lung specimens. Arch Pathol Lab Med. 2005;129(12):1602–1609.

Soares FA. Increased numbers of pulmonary megakaryocytes in patients with arterial pulmonary tumour embolism and lung metastases seen at necropsy. J Clin Pathol. 1992;45:140–142.

Flieder DB. Commonly encountered difficulties in pathologic staging of lung cancer. Arch Pathol Lab Med 2007;131:1016–1026.

Kutla CA, Urer N, Olgac G. Carcinoma in situ from the view of complete resection. Lung Cancer 2004;46:383–385.

Marchevsky AM, Changsri C, Gupta I, et al. Frozen section diagnoses of small pulmonary nodules: accuracy and clinical implications. Ann Thorac Surg 2004;78:1755–1759.

Massard G, Doddoli C, Gassar B, et al. Prognostic implications of a positive bronchial resection margin. Eur J Cardiothorac Surg 2000;17:557–565.

Maygarden SJ, Detterbeck FC, Funkhouser WK. Bronchial margins in lung cancer resection specimens: utility of frozen section and gross evaluation. Mod Pathol 2004;17:1080–1086.

Sienko A, Allen TC, Zander D, Cagle PT. Frozen section of lung specimens. Arch Pathol Lab Med 2005;129:1602–1609.

Sirmali M, Demirag F, Turut H, et al. Utility of intraoperative frozen section examination in thoracic surgery. A review of 721 cases. Cardiovasc Surg (Torino) 2006;47:83–87.

Snijder RJ, Brutel de la Riviere A, Elbers HJ, van den Bosch JM. Survival in resected stage I lung cancer with residual tumor at the bronchial resection margin. Ann Thorac Surg 1998;65:212–216.

Thunnissen FB, den Bakker MA. Implications of frozen section analyses from bronchial resection margins in NSCLC. Histopathology 2005;47:638–640.

Index

Printed in the United States